D0960250

CLEAN

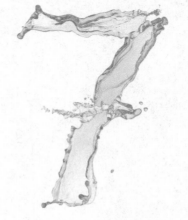

Supercharge the Body's Natural Ability to Heal Itself—

THE ONE-WEEK BREAKTHROUGH
DETOX PROGRAM

CLEAN

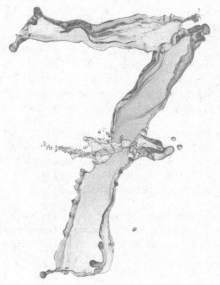

7

ALEJANDRO JUNGER, MD
WITH RECIPES BY CHEF JAMES BARRY

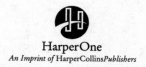

HarperOne
An Imprint of HarperCollinsPublishers

HarperOne

This book contains advice and information relating to health care. It should be used to supplement rather than replace the advice of your doctor or another trained health professional. If you know or suspect you have a health problem, it is recommended that you seek your physician's advice before embarking on any medical program or treatment. All efforts have been made to assure the accuracy of the information contained in this book as of the date of publication. This publisher and the author disclaim liability for any medical outcomes that may occur as a result of applying the methods suggested in this book.

HarperCollins books may be purchased for educational, business, or sales promotional use. For information, please email the Special Markets Department at SPsales@harpercollins.com.

FIRST EDITION

Designed by Diahann Sturge

Library of Congress Cataloging-in-Publication Data is available upon request.

ISBN 978-0-06-279228-0
ISBN 978-0-06-298998-7 (Intl)

19 20 21 22 23 LSC 10 9 8 7 6 5 4 3 2 1

I dedicate this book to my parents.
To Muky, my mama, whose love knows no limits,
and to Beilo, my papa, who still guides me from above.
I miss him every day of my life.

Contents

FOREWORD BY ANTHONY WILLIAM, THE MEDICAL MEDIUM   ix

INTRODUCTION   1

1   What Is CLEAN7?   7

2   The Three Pillars of CLEAN7   22

3   Getting Ready for CLEAN7   56

4   The CLEAN7 Program Day by Day   83

5   Detox Your Mind by Becoming Present   108

6   As Above, So Below: CLEAN Meets ORGANIC INDIA   123

7   Now What?   136

The CLEAN7 Tools   143

Your CLEAN7 Planner   145

The CLEAN Diet: The Complete List   154

Find Your Dosha Questionnaire   156

Chart 1: Vata Dosha Foods to Enjoy and Foods to Avoid   158

Chart 2: Pitta Dosha Foods to Enjoy and Foods to Avoid   160

Chart 3: Kapha Dosha Foods to Enjoy and Foods to Avoid   162

Chart 4: Combined Elimination Diet
    and Vata Dosha Foods to Enjoy and Foods to Avoid   164

Chart 5: Combined Elimination Diet
    and Pitta Dosha Foods to Enjoy and Foods to Avoid   168

Chart 6: Combined Elimination Diet
    and Kapha Dosha Foods to Enjoy and Foods to Avoid   172

Other Ways to Follow Through after Doing CLEAN7   176

Detox Your Life   179

The CLEAN7 Kitchen and Recipes   185

Introduction to the CLEAN7 Recipes   187

Vata Recipes   194

Pitta Recipes   220

Kapha Recipes   245

Celebratory Meals   272

ACKNOWLEDGMENTS   285

BIBLIOGRAPHY   287

INDEX   291

Foreword by
Anthony William, the Medical Medium

There is a secret epidemic right now. As you read this, there are over a billion people suffering with some chronic illness or symptom. You might be one of them. *Chronic illness* isn't a term just for those who are gravely ill and unable to function. If you have acne, eczema, migraines, fatigue, blood sugar issues, mood swings, brain fog, tingles and numbness, bloating, urinary tract infections, anxiety, depression, constipation, or any other symptom or illness that recurs or is long lasting, it means you too are among those who have a chronic illness or symptom. Most people have become so accustomed to living life with a symptom or hearing about the symptoms and conditions family and friends live with that chronic illness has become a normal part of life. But living with symptoms and illnesses isn't normal. It is not natural. It's not how you were meant to live. There's only one way we can curtail the epidemic of chronic illness that is growing at an alarming rate: we must remember that chronic illness and symptoms are not a normal part of life and actively seek answers to what is causing them and how they can be healed.

One of the greatest barriers to healing we are facing today is that medical research and science don't know the root causes of most chronic illnesses and symptoms. How can people suffering with a chronic illness get the answers they need to truly heal from within the medical system? The truth is that they can't. This is one of the main reasons the epidemic of chronic illness is growing so rapidly.

Over the decades I have witnessed many thousands of people who have been failed by the limitations of the medical system and medical research and science. This is through no fault of the hardworking, caring, highly intelligent doctors, surgeons, nurses, and other medical professionals who have devoted themselves to saving people's lives and trying to help the sick and injured. I have great respect for these selfless individuals. They provide critical care if you're in a car accident, your appendix bursts, you break your ankle, and so much more. There is no question that modern medicine saves lives and that we would be in peril without it. But when it comes to chronic illness, research and science are sadly still in the dark ages, and doctors and other medical professionals have only the information medical research and science provides them with. Patients are typically offered only surgery and/or medication and are very often turned away without real answers as to why they are suffering, even if they receive a diagnosis.

At some point, every doctor, surgeon, and medical professional is faced with the limitations of science. When yet one more patient, family member, or friend is *still* suffering, and no surgery or medication is helping, or when their own health is declining, it raises the question for open-minded and forward-thinking doctors: is there more than what medical research and science can offer us? This is the question Dr. Alejandro Junger found himself asking when his own health was challenged and he couldn't find any answers or a way out of his suffering within the medical system, despite all of his education, training, connections, and experience. He witnessed one person after another having the same defeating experience he was having and being presented with only surgery or medication as treatment options, neither of which offer true, long-lasting healing for so many. His intuition, compassion, and reason told him there must be more to discover—more answers, more healing, more truth. He saw in nature that chronic illness didn't exist for animals to the degree it does for humans and asked himself where the human species was going wrong. Why were so many people so sick?

In his search for answers, Dr. Junger explored many healing modalities outside of the medical model he was trained in. Despite already being at the top of his game, he wasn't content to stick with the status quo. He continually went above and beyond because of his desire to see people heal. His wholehearted exploration led him to realize a fundamental healing truth: the foods we eat and the medicinal properties we receive from herbs and other plants have the power to heal us in ways that research and science haven't yet discovered. It is in their infinite, secret intelligence that we can uncover healing. This is a topic that is near and dear to my heart and that stands front and center in all the healing information I share because I know that the right foods have the power to change lives when used correctly. Dr. Junger tapped into this transformational truth, and it became deeply entrenched in his soul. He has dedicated his life's work since this discovery to helping people heal by harnessing the innate powers of the foods available to us on this planet.

One of the great misconceptions today is that the most recent generations of people will live longer than the generations before them. This was true at one point, but times are quickly changing and this is no longer the case. Dr. Junger speaks about this in *CLEAN7*. The lifespan of each generation is about to become shorter and shorter due to the degree of toxins and pathogens—and the resulting sicknesses—we are up against. This trajectory isn't going to change unless humankind reads a book such as this, learns from it, puts its advice into practice, and holds onto it for generations to come. Our future on Earth can hold promise only if we have the opportunity to experience good enough health and long enough lives to do what we feel we are here to do. And this can happen only if we possess the wisdom we need.

When I read the pages of Dr. Alejandro Junger's book, I witness the wisdom inside. I see the great hope it provides for generation upon generation to start living longer and healthier lives. Dr. Junger knows the world is a toxic place and yet we have to live here. We can't just ignore the truth that our bodies are under siege from toxins. But knowing the world is full of toxins—and so too our bodies— is only valuable if you possess something of greater importance: the knowledge of how to remove the toxins and poisons that we absorb every day and how to support our body's self-healing ability. It is our right to know how to be free from the symptoms that plague us and slow us down.

CLEAN7 is about the importance of detoxing. Whether it's poisons from toxic, processed foods we eat or chemicals we are exposed to on a daily basis, it's critical to know how to start lightening the toxic load. I ask myself, is there anything more important than helping provide a healthier life for the chronically ill—in fact, for anyone? And I ask you, does how you feel matter to you? What about how your loved ones feel? These questions are worthy because you are worthy. Your loved ones are worthy. Everyone on planet Earth is here for a reason. You matter. Your loved ones matter. You deserve to be healthy and feel your best, and to do so you need the health wisdom that can get you there. Dr. Junger knows you deserve the best opportunity to heal and has committed his life to helping you do so.

I have been blessed to connect with many amazing doctors, surgeons, and other medical professionals over my lifetime. I greatly respect and revere all the doctors and professionals who genuinely care about their patients and want to look after their best interests. But when I first met Dr. Junger I knew he was one of the special ones. His devotion to his patients, community, friends, and family was obvious. His genuine and kind nature was apparent in the way he talked about his work and the people he felt moved to help. His quest for truth had led him to search the world over for answers that could change people's lives. Dr. Junger's heart of gold and desire to be of service stood out and still does today. He is a man of compassion, a brilliant doctor with integrity, and a leader in the health and wellness world. He has a powerful ability to see through the darkness of suffering and guide those seeking freedom from sickness to safe ground. He truly cares about the souls who struggle with their health. It's a great honor to be one of the first to read through the pages of his book. I know Dr. Junger has written *CLEAN7* with the intent of helping you to step closer to the healthy life that is your birthright. I know he wants you to be free of the symptoms and illnesses so many people are suffering from today. I am thankful to Dr. Junger for being the compassionate doctor and author that he is. He is truly a bright light for healing on this planet.

ANTHONY WILLIAM, THE MEDICAL MEDIUM

Introduction

I spent the end-of-year holidays with my kids in Todos Santos, Baja California Sur. The whales were arriving from feeding in the cold waters of Alaska to mate in the warmer lagoons of Mexico. The spectacle was amazing. We saw them breaching all day long, and the kids were in heaven. They love nature. We joined a sea turtle rescue mission that protects eggs from beach tourism and releases the baby turtles at sundown, clearing their path in the sand so they can walk all the way to the shoreline and be swallowed by the ocean. Beilo, my eight-year-old son, and Fina, my six-year-old daughter, had so many questions. "That's not very smart, it's so hard for them to walk all that distance," said Beilo. "Papa, why don't we just put them in the ocean directly?" Hearing the question, the rescue team chief answered, "It is better for them to walk all the way on their own. That is how they remember many years from now where to come back to lay their own eggs. Those are the rules."

They both turned to me and Fina asked, "Who made the rules, Papa?" "Nature made the rules," I answered. "Nature designed planet Earth and all the animals on it, which includes you both and all humans. And nature is incredibly smart. Not only does it help the turtles come back to this spot to lay eggs or the whales to swim all the way from Alaska to have babies here, but nature also helped you guys grow in mama's belly and helped you come out when you were ready. The rules of nature are what makes every-thing work well at the same time, all the time, without forgetting about anything. That is how nature makes sure that all animals live a good healthy life." Without missing a beat, Beilo asked, "But then why do people get sick? Did nature forget about us?" I like to think that my kids are geniuses, but hanging out with their friends made me realize that most kids are. Here was my eight-year-old son asking the most important question about health, one that I did not start asking myself until I was in my thirties, even years after becoming a doctor: why do we get sick? Did Nature forget about us? I put my arms around my kids and answered, "Humans don't get sick because nature forgot about us. We get sick because humans forgot about nature."

Why do people get sick? The answer to this question created a profound shift in how I view medicine and treat patients. I went to medical school to learn what healthy cells look like and how to detect sick ones. I learned how the body works and the ways in which a good medical history, examination, and laboratory tests can reveal and confirm where and what the problems are. I was soon able to identify the different diseases by name and prescribe a treatment plan for each. I got so carried away studying the *how* that I forgot to ask the *why*. After medical school I started my train-ing in hospitals, where the rubber meets the road. I had to apply everything I had learned in classrooms to helping people in real life.

After three years of internal medicine I chose cardiology for another three years of training. As most doctors will tell you, this training is grueling. Endless days and sleepless nights. I wouldn't have slowed down if it weren't for the fact that I got really sick. After consulting three specialists (an allergist, a gastroenterologist, and a psychiatrist), I was given three diagnoses; severe allergies, irritable bowel syndrome, and severe depression. Between the various doctors, I was prescribed seven medications, including antidepressants, anxiolytics, anti-allergics, antidiarrheals, and antispasmodics. My career race had come to a screeching halt. Almost immediately, I couldn't function without pills. And the worst part of it was that I didn't even want to. I knew, however, that this wasn't normal. This wasn't natural. Finally, a few months later the big question popped into my head again: Why did I get sick? *Why*?

Even though the treatment I was prescribed was in line with what I had learned in medical school, in all my years of hospital training, and it was what I was offering all my patients, when it came to following that advice myself, a pill for each one of my symptoms did not make sense. My intuition told me to reject taking pills. They weren't healing as much as silencing symptoms by forcing a certain chemistry on my body. This realization changed the course of my life and my medical practice for good.

I began to search for ways to get healthy—to feel well—that did not include medications. I looked everywhere for answers. I didn't know exactly what I was looking for or where to find it, so I kept trying different things. My search took me around the world. I discovered that I needed to rethink modern medicine in the context of healing and that part of it meant opening my mind to learning from ancient systems. I found new tools in different places and eventually understood exactly why I got sick, and more importantly, what I needed to do about it. The pivotal moment in my health came when I discovered the concepts and practices of detoxification. After completing a well-designed detoxification program, not only was I able to rid myself of all my symptoms, but also felt and looked ten years younger. My body had restored its optimal functioning. I was, briefly put, rejuvenated. After this discovery, I have never stopped looking for other healing tools, both new and ancient. My mission has remained constant: to help people better understand the body's natural ability to heal itself. I have discovered that there is in fact a single common underlying principle in every proven healing practice: these methods all help the human body better align itself with nature. Nature's incredible intelligence is embedded in all living organisms and when its rules are respected it results in vibrant health. Animals that live in the places where nature designed them to live and eat what nature designed them to eat rarely get chronic diseases. In the wild, bears don't get depressed, alligators don't get diabetes, eagles don't get cancer. We are the only species on the planet that is unwell most of the time.

I wrote *CLEAN7* to share the answers I found when asking why so many of us are sick and how breaking the laws of nature is at the heart of today's epidemic of chronic diseases. This book will teach you how to use some of the most powerful healing tools in the world to shed your own chronic symptoms and illnesses and finally live the life you were meant to live. These tools have already improved the lives of millions of patients worldwide for millennia. My goal in writing this book is to make this health transformation more accessible and easier to implement than ever before.

It doesn't matter if you are just starting your path to a healthier you or if you are way ahead on the road; the principles and practices in this book can take you to the next level and help you stay there for the long run.

If your life has been busy and your health has taken a back seat, this is the perfect way to start. I'll take away any confusion you may have felt when browsing the complex world of current lifestyle options and programs available. With CLEAN7, this no longer needs to be the case. This seven-day program is user-friendly and incredibly effective. The foods to eat, the supplements to take, the practices and the protocol necessary to implement this life-changing program are spelled out day by day and hour by hour. I will hold your hand on this health journey and make sure that you meet your desired goals. Whether you are wrestling with your weight, your mood, your energy, mild symptoms, or chronic symptoms, I promise you that by the end of seven days, this program will change your perspective on what is possible for you. You will feel better than you have in a long time, and you will learn tools for maintaining lifelong lasting health.

If you are a pro, already have found a lifestyle that fits you, and are doing great, CLEAN7 will help you stay there or go even further. The ideas in this book will help you connect the dots regarding things that you may already be doing but were not quite sure why they work.

My dear reader, all I ask is a week of your time for a health revolution that will last you a lifetime.

Welcome to CLEAN7.

1

What Is CLEAN7?

CLEAN7 is a seven-day detox program designed to jumpstart the process of restoring your body's natural ability to heal itself. It is based on core principles from three sources: (1) Functional Medicine, (2) Ayurvedic Medicine, and (3) intermittent fasting. On their own, each one of these practices is a powerful tool for recalibrating the body and mind, restoring the natural and intended functioning of your bodily systems, thus reversing and preventing symptomatic dysfunction. What I found by integrating tools from all three into one easy-to-follow program is incredible. Combined, the three are an unstoppable, powerful force that will guide you to a new understanding of what it means to be healthy. I think of it as the yoga of detox. The word *yoga* in Sanskrit means union. CLEAN7 is the union of both modern and ancient sciences. Just as yoga achieves its balancing results by activating and recalibrating nervous pathways through physical movements, the CLEAN7 program will bring physiologic balance by activating and recalibrating your inner chemistry, moving nutrients, antioxidants, and Ayurvedic adaptogenic herbs through your blood.

From Functional Medicine, I draw on the science that addresses the overload of toxicity. Simply put, this field has studied the ways in which the body is damaged by the dangerous amount of toxins we are exposed to in our day-to-day lives. I will detail the chemicals to which you are exposed, how to remove them from your diet and life, and, ultimately, how to nutritionally support your body's detox processes to empower your cells and organs to do their work of detoxification.

From Ayurvedic Medicine, I tap into to an ancient healing system that considers detox as the necessary beginning to any healing plan. Ayurveda has proven to have effective tools for reversing disease, as well as for activating and accelerating cellular rejuvenation. One of Ayurveda's powerful tools is identifying your body's constitution or type, what is known as your dosha, as a way to personalize your healing process. It guides you to avoid foods that slow down your body's ability to detoxify and repair. Also following Ayurvedic Medicine principles, I bring in Ayurvedic herbs not only to provide incredibly bioavailable nutrients and antioxidants but also to energetically turbocharge the detox and healing processes.

From the research on intermittent fasting CLEAN7 borrows the understanding of how to recreate the inner conditions in which our genes will shift their work from activating adaptation and survival mechanisms to one of generating vibrancy and balance. This, in turn, translates into vital hormonal and metabolic shifts that help you restore optimal function and repair the body.

The effect is a radical shift in the way you look and feel. In just seven days, you will break through the "wellness paralysis" that so many of us fall into. I define this as the state of confusion so many of my patients experience because of the excess of information surrounding health and wellness available to them. The fluctuating cultural narrative about what to eat, how much to eat, and when to eat creates uncertainty, and so many are left unable to take the first and most important step toward a healthy lifestyle. I wrote this book to bridge this gap and to offer a short and simple program that is easy to follow. Everything you need to know is in these pages and within one week you will not only feel amazing, look better, be mentally sharper, but you will also have a better understanding of which foods work best for you and which foods work against you. And you will be able to discover this for yourself without expensive and often inaccurate food allergy tests. CLEAN7 is the health jump-start that you have been waiting for.

Imagine a person who hasn't bathed for years. The dirt and sweat have combined to encase the skin, not letting it breathe. The odor extends a few feet around, there's no avoiding it. Since the smell has accumulated slowly for years, that person is probably so used to it that the smell is not bothersome. The overgrown nails store yet more dirt. The overgrown hair is greasy and entangled. There is not even a memory of what being clean looks or feels like.

Now imagine this person taking a warm shower, followed by a long, hot bath, soaked in aromatic salts and soaps, oils and scrubs. After that, a hair wash, brushing, and trim. And then a mani-pedi. What would that person feel and look like? This is what CLEAN7 can do for your cells, and that is how your cleaner cells will make you feel—and how they'll make you look.

For those of you already on the path of a health journey, I have designed this program to work as your companion, one that might evolve with you and help you in that quest. It doesn't matter if you follow a vegetarian, vegan, paleo, keto, or macrobiotic lifestyle, CLEAN7 will enhance your body's detox ability and make whatever you are already doing work better.

I believe it is crucial for all of us to learn about our body's detoxification abilities. CLEAN7 provides this understanding by sharing the tools that will serve you for the rest of your life. The book is the culmination of over thirty years of education, practice, and research. Like so many doctors, I was "detox blind." The few times I heard anything about it I thought of it as a new age trend, that there was no real science behind it. Later, desperately looking for solutions to my own health problems, I found them in detox. By that time, many celebrities were talking about detox, which brought on a wave of criticism and labeling anything detox related as a "celebrity fad." This has prevented countless chronically ill people from benefiting from the detox revolution. I want to set the record straight.

MUCH OF DETOX'S reputational blowback comes from a culture unwilling to acknowledge the degree to which the toxins in the air, the water, and our food are affecting our health. The vast majority of people who work in mainstream medicine have not studied the research or seen firsthand the results that can be achieved through aiding the body's detoxification systems. Their belief is that toxicity and our exposure to it has been overblown by a bunch of alternative healers simply trying to make a buck. And as with most professions, there are always a few bad apples. That said, most of my colleagues who use detox programs as pillars of their practice are dedicated, responsible, brilliant doctors whose primary goal and mission is to help patients heal. We are on the frontlines seeing patients suffering and looking for answers. We have seen, studied, and tested the results of doctor-managed detoxification programs. We know that they can both reverse and prevent a myriad of symptoms and diseases.

Personally, after experiencing the powerful results of detoxing, studying the subject deeply, and guiding thousands of people through detox programs, I am 100 percent convinced that detoxification programs are a powerful and ever more necessary healing tool for people all over the planet. That said, a detox program alone won't solve every problem. What you do with it makes all the difference. If in our example above a person finally bathing and grooming after eons of being dirty goes back to doing exactly as before, the dirt and all its consequences will return soon. But after feeling *so good*, no one would want to go back. This is my hope when you do the CLEAN7 program. At minimum, it can be like a detox shower you take every so often so you never go back to constantly feeling unwell. At its best, it can totally transform your health so you never look back at your nagging, symptom-ridden past life. It will take a while for detox to become mainstream as something that most doctors will guide their patients through periodically. There are many opinions and institutions that play a role in how and when such shifts in paradigm become mainstream. There are big financial interests in things remaining the same. Nevertheless, there are ideas and practices that have survived for thousands of years, and they appear in waves throughout generations. There is nothing stronger than an idea whose time has come, again. The wave of detox is growing, and for good reason. It is time for you to surf the detox wave without waiting for official institutional approval of a consciousness shift that is already sweeping the planet.

FAD vs. FDA

During my medical training, I was taught to follow the Food and Drug Administration's (FDA) approved treatments. Sets of agreements and approvals from academic and government organizations, including the FDA, heavily regulate standard medical practice and the legal implications of treating patients. This is important because many of modern medicine's treatments are risky, especially when misused, but even when correctly prescribed. The problem is that later people get confused about what is medically approved, what is scientifically proven, what is standard medical practice, and which recent medical research results have been given the wrong attention. Many people follow instructions simply because they are presented as results of the latest medical research. The term *medical research* is used to refer to different things, from double-blind placebo-controlled experiments that go through peer review to someone just gathering information to explain a theory. Furthermore, not everything that the medical community advises is correct, even if it has been backed up by research and FDA approval. And often what becomes the consensus shifts over time, leading to whole new ways of doing things. Many trends are based on research, but many are not, and even incorrect ideas find support in research. It happens all the time. Sometimes it happens because research results are rigged or because the study was not designed or interpreted properly. And so, a roller coaster of discoveries, trial results, trends, and fads shift entire industries. Even worse, they set up what becomes perceived as standard medical practice.

When the news is generated by doctors, it gathers force fast. Sometimes it lingers even when disproven. Just think of what happened in the United States over the last fifty years or so regarding fat and carbohydrates. First, we started the war on carbs. Low-carb versions of everything appeared in the shelves of every supermarket. Carbs became the mortal enemy, even a social taboo. But after a decade we decided we had the wrong enemy and fat became the bad guy. Food manufacturers quickly shifted course. Nobody talked about low carb any longer as no-fat and low-fat products invaded the supermarket shelves. Oh boy, how things have changed—again! America is falling in love with fat. In fact, we are on a "fat honeymoon." Eating fat now seems to be the solution for all problems. The fat-loving diets such as Atkins, paleo, and keto are all enjoying a renewed boost in public awareness. Yet, many old school doctors keep talking about fat as the enemy, regardless of whether it is plant fat or animal fat, a "good" fat or a "bad" fat. And that is why it is vital for doctors and medical professionals to keep an open mind as they continue to research ways to help alleviate the issues raised by patients. They continue to learn more every day, and very often this knowledge is recovered from the past.

The Oxymoron of an "Ancient Fad"

The concepts and practices around detox are not new; in fact, they are thousands of years old. Entire systems of medicine were built around detox as one of the main pillars of health and longevity, long before the tsunami of toxins that is drowning us today. These ancient systems, such as Ayurvedic and Chinese medicine, have for centuries been proven incredibly effective. There is nothing "short lived," as stated in the definition of the word *fad*, about detox. Jokingly, it is perhaps the world's longest clinical trial. Seriously, while modern medicine has all the knowledge of the different detox processes from a cellular and molecular point of view, it wasn't until Functional Medicine combined ancient knowledge with modern science that the connections between the dysfunctions of the detox systems and the resulting chronic health issues were made clear. My colleagues and I soon discovered that detoxification programs were the best tool available to successfully treat many of the ailments caused by the overload of toxins we are experiencing. The results have been staggering and detoxification has positively impacted the health and lives of millions of individuals.

Detox Means What?

I never heard the use of the word *detox* in medical school outside of the subject of addictions. Alcoholics and addicts to other drugs were sent to detox programs. *Toxicity* was used only as a synonym for *poisoning* and we learned about it when studying certain dangerous chemicals, as well as animal and plant poisons to which the local population could be accidentally exposed. In other words, we learned about the problems that could possibly appear in our emergency rooms.

Of course, we studied the different organs involved in detoxification and their functions in detail, but never spoke about toxicity and detoxification programs as something that we should regularly consider, evaluate the need for, and help people perform. Our professors spoke of endogenous toxins—meaning generated in the body—as the toxic waste products of cellular metabolism. Many of these are only detected when their accumulation in blood becomes extreme and therefore extreme measures are needed to treat it. For example, kidney function is measured by testing the blood levels of creatinine, a waste product of the continuous muscle breakdown in our bodies. Creatinine starts accumulating abnormally only after more than 80 percent of both kidneys fail, which is often too late to reverse the chronic condition that caused the kidneys to fail. Dialysis, as extreme a measure as it is, does the work of the kidneys and keeps people alive. As students, we also studied exogenous toxins—meaning coming from outside the body—aka xenobiotics, substances that are foreign to the body and act as pollutants or poisons. We never considered or discussed all the chemicals we consume daily in our food as exogenous toxins. We saw everything as just food. So, when Functional Medicine practitioners discuss detoxification, we aren't making up the medical science. The truth is that understanding the "detox program" concept is just a matter of looking at what we already know from a different perspective.

Do We Need to Detox?

Our comfortable modern lifestyle stresses our bodies and, to different degrees, we are all suffering the consequences. Almost no one's body functions optimally anymore. The majority of us have health issues, whether they are minor symptoms such as headaches, bloating, bad breath, constipation, sleep difficulties, thinning hair, brittle nails, puffy skin, poor digestion, acidity, nagging aches and pains, or more chronic diseases such as diabetes, cancer, autoimmune disease, heart disease, and depression. The minor symptoms often don't add up to anything scary enough to warrant seeing a doctor. And even if we do decide to consult a physician, most doctors don't look for the root causes of our symptoms. We end up taking over-the-counter medications and getting on with our busy life. For chronic issues, we go to the doctor and most of the time we get a prescription pill for each ill or undergo surgery. As disease statistics continue to rise across the board, doctors around the world scratch their heads. How did we get here? Doctors are doing what they are trained to do—fighting illness one issue at a time. As individuals and patients, our collective choices feel limited: take pills to mask the symptoms, ignoring the underlying cause, cut pieces off your body, or suffer. Despite the onslaught of poor health, most of us are not taking a preventive approach and even less looking for a natural approach. This has become the fate of our bodies in the world today. We live with anxiety. We live with diabetes. We live with IBS. This is not how it is meant to be. This is not natural.

In the introduction, I spoke about the fact that animals living in nature don't get chronically sick. Elephants aren't walking around with a host of perpetual nagging symptoms like headaches or constipation. What is it about human life that is so unnatural? It is difficult to answer this question with any perspective because we take life as it is today for granted. We explain the difference in our lifestyle to animals within the context of modernization. We are grateful that we don't live in the wild, escaping from tigers, and constantly looking for food. The way we live is all we truly know. It is our "normal" and we don't question it. Primitive cultures that have survived the modern revolution live way more in line with nature, but we typically think of them as unevolved, lingering fragments of history long past. Thankfully, scientists have been paying more attention after noticing that these primitive cultures, if they remain isolated, don't suffer from many of the problems we have in modern industrialized societies.

We are misled by the fact that until recently we were living longer than the generation before us. "We must be doing something right if that is the case" many argue. But it looks like the latest generations will start living shorter lives than those of their parents. We have created a world in which we are constantly bombarded by toxins. These unnatural substances surround us and enter our bodies through the air we breathe, the water we drink, and the food we consume. The problem is that our bodies cannot keep up with today's abnormally higher demand for the constant process of detoxification necessary to maintain optimal function. On top of the abnormally high amounts of toxins, at a moment when detox should be even more efficient, the lack of nutrients necessary to detox slows down and blocks many of the detox pathways. The good news is that our bodies are built with the ability to combat these substances and we can help the body's natural detoxification processes. This is what CLEAN7 is all about.

With all the information available today, why is it that we have not figured out how to live truly healthy, vibrant lives? It is about time that we all get up to speed on what detox really is and why it is important. It is imperative that we all learn how to support our detox organs and systems as well as minimize the exposure to toxins so that in the future we don't have to periodically do "detox programs." As life is today though, detox programs may be the difference between vibrant health and a gradual accumulation of minor symptoms that in time add up to a disease, or many diseases, that will zap you out of the life that you want. CLEAN7 is the program I needed back when I was contemplating taking seven medications several times a day just to function.

The Bad News

It is not my intention to scare you when you read the next paragraphs, but fear is inevitable. What I'm about to say is all over the news, and you have most likely heard much of it in different places. But when you hear it all at once, it's ugly. My work would not be complete if I sugarcoated the story, though. You need to know the big picture, and when you do, you will get scared. I promise to help you transform that fear into a plan of action, however, which will not only take away the fear but will allow you to escape the inevitable suffering that will come from ignoring what I am about to tell you.

If you live in a typical American house, even if you get a good eight hours of sleep at night, your body is probably hard at work defending itself from toxic chemicals you just don't think of and never heard about. Your mattress most likely contains fire retardants and other chemicals. As your sheets, pillowcases, and pajamas have been rubbing against your skin, so has the residue of the detergents, softeners, and scents with which you washed them. You step out of bed and walk barefoot on your hardwood floors or your cozy carpets. Chances are they are off-gassing benzene, 4-phenylcyclohexane (4-PC) used to make carpet backing, or the solvent perchloroethylene (PERC), all known carcinogens. In the bathroom, you splash water onto your face or get under the shower. Most city-supplied water contains all kinds of unwanted and unintended toxic chemicals, as well as some intended ones: trihalomethanes (THMs) such as chloroform, chlorine, and lead—and just about every medication you can imagine, including antidepressants, erectile dysfunction meds, anti-inflammatories, and antibiotics. You then squeeze some toothpaste onto your toothbrush, and with it, sodium lauryl sulfate (SLS), which is a foaming agent, the antibacterial triclosan, and the artificial sweetener aspartame. If you wear makeup, your moisturizer, foundation, eye shadow, mascara, eyeliner, and lipstick are likely loaded with molecules such as parabens and phthalates, both of which are endocrine disrupters. You don't want to offend others at work, so you soak your armpits with deodorant probably filled with aluminum; propylene glycol (a form of alcohol used in antifreeze!); triethanolamine (TEA), which is produced by mixing ammonia with ethylene; and diethanolamine (DEA), on the list of hazardous substances because it is corrosive.

Your favorite part of the day is about to start, and you are salivating already. Bacon, eggs, cereal with milk, fruit, and coffee. Breakfast, yum. As it all fills your tummy, it turns into a smoothie of sorts. If you buy processed foods, it will be a toxic smoothie full of nitrates, sodium erythorbate nitrosamines, arsenic, antibiotics, organochlorine pesticides, glyphosate, butylated hydroxyanisole (BHA), butylated hydroxytoluene (BHT), the pesticide DDT—yes, it is still in the environment, antimony carbaryl (another pesticide), ochratoxin A (a mycotoxin produced by certain fungi), bisphenol A (BPA), acrylamides (potentially toxic and possibly cancer-causing chemicals), bovine growth hormone (rBGH), perchlorate (a naturally occurring and manufactured chemical that is a known hormone disrupter), and antibiotics.

Before you get to work you are exposed to hundreds, if not thousands, of chemicals that alone or in combination are known to cause all kinds of symptoms and are linked to chronic diseases. And this is your safe space, your home. Once you enter your workplace a new tsunami of toxic chemicals washes over you in little and big waves all day long. Until you get back home, where it starts all over again. No other animal is exposed to this constant barrage of assaults, except for our domestic animals. They live in our houses and eat food-like products too, just like we do, and they also get sick like we do: dogs and cats can develop diabetes, cancer, allergies, and obesity, all the same chronic diseases that we suffer from. When sick, humans and domestic animals alike ingest painkillers, antidepressants, decongestants, anti-inflammatories, and antibiotics, all of which present yet another massive insult to our biology. The active ingredients in medications are a life saver for many, but this is not all you are swallowing with the pills, which are also loaded with fillers, excipients, dyes, and many other potentially toxic chemicals used for shape, hardness, color, solubility and even taste. I have recently been educated by the founders of Genexa, a company that makes over-the-counter meds without *any* toxic chemicals, just the active ingredients and when necessary, organic nontoxic components. I am still shocked at the amounts and variety of toxic chemicals that I learned are in our medications. This information is not yet widely available, but the cat is out of the bag. Especially when it involves my children, this can be very scary. The most famous brand of acetaminophen, which every parent I know uses for fevers, contains so many potentially toxic ingredients, many that are associated with allergies and other toxic effects. Some of these are high-fructose corn syrup, FD&C red #40, aluminum lake, Hypromellose, magnesium stearate, carboxymeth-ylcellulose, propylene glycol, and sucralose. Compare this with Genexa's acetaminophen ingredient list: acetaminophen, organic agave, organic flavor, and organic citrus preservative. Which one would you use for your kids? Learn more at www.genexa.com.

The Cumulative Effect

The air we breathe, the water we drink and bathe in, the cosmetics and body products we use, the detergents we clean everything with, the medications we take, our kitchen utensils, and mostly the foods we eat, are loaded with toxic chemicals that alone or in combina-tion cause all kinds of dysfunctions that lead to chronic symptoms. In time, these symptoms develop into full-blown diseases, many of them deadly, but even in the best-case scenario, they steal the state of ease, wellness, vitality, and happiness that is your birthright.

I know, it's bad. This is scientifically proven, serious stuff. Toxins and toxicity are not just vague words that snake oil salesmen use to scare people. These Persistent Organic Pollutants (POPs) are real molecules, exposure to which causes dysfunction and imbalance in the body and leads to disease. On top of the toxic barrage the human body is subjected to day in and day out, we are unknowingly slowing down and interfering with its biotransformation, the cellular activ-ity that transforms a toxic molecule into a nontoxic one, within the detoxification organs and systems. In the world in which we live, we need these systems to work effectively and at top speed, now more than ever. Despite this, we are creating obstacles and not providing what the body needs to do what it knows how to do, and is in fact desperate to do. And as long as our detoxification systems are not supported, toxins will accumulate, the body will try to adapt and defend itself, and everything will be thrown out of balance. Global toxicity is the most unnatural phenomenon; it interferes with nature's organizing intelligence and is why so many of us get sick.

The Good News

Your body already knows how to rid itself of toxins and it knows how to repair the damage they might have caused. What is *not* true is that our bodies are always able to do that job effectively. An overload of toxins and lack of detox essential nutrients can interfere with the complex chemical reactions needed to render both endogenous and exogenous toxins harmless and water soluble so they can be eliminated via breath, sweat, urine, and feces. Digestion, inflammation, allergies, sensitivities, hormonal imbalances, and lack of sleep also divert or steal energy from our detox systems.

Once we begin to address these issues by supporting the detox systems, the chemical reactions of toxin-biotransformation will happen effectively. Your liver cells, and others, will identify the molecules that cause trouble and get to work on them through a series of enzymatic reactions such as sulfation, methylation, glucuronidation, and others. When the right conditions are created, everything runs like clockwork, with the result that toxicity can be contained and reduced enough to achieve vibrant health.

Detox is not a fad. It is real. It is the fundamental pillar for some of the most ancient systems of medicine and has been proven beneficial over millennia. We now understand it better than ever from a medical, biological, biochemical, and physiological point of view, and thanks to Functional Medicine we are able to think of it from a systems perspective. We also now understand detoxing better from a psychological, emotional, and spiritual point of view, thanks to ancient medical systems, such as Ayurveda. Furthermore, we now know how to accelerate and strengthen the detox processes through another practice that has also been around for thousands of years but had been put aside until recently due to the lack of scientific understanding of it. I am talking about intermittent fasting.

In the following chapters I will explain the principles upon which the CLEAN7 program is based and how I learned about them. Then I will guide you day by day on how to complete the program. Finally, I will explain what to do after you finish the week's program and how you can use CLEAN7 as a powerful tool to regain and maintain your well-being, evolving with you in the future.

The tools that make up the CLEAN7 program have been used independently by many, but have never before been combined into an easy-to-follow program. The result is a synergistic boost that potentiates what you can achieve to levels that make the results so much deeper and faster. There are no limitations to what nature can do; the limitations are only in our understanding, which guides what we do. The more alignment with nature, the more its power is unleashed, healing being one of those powers that remains partly hidden to our understanding. The next chapter will give you some of the intellectual understanding of how it all works but doing the program will give you the cellular experience of how it feels when nature is deploying its full intelligence, unobstructed and at full speed, the way nature designed it and intended it to be.

Many people think of medicine as science. Some people think of medicine as art. I think of medicine as art restoration, with the patient as art and nature as the artist. When restoring a work of art, it is important to know about the medium, technique, brushes, and paints used to create the art and even ask yourself, what would the artist do?

When I practice medicine I often ask myself, what would nature do? CLEAN7 is the perfect restoration start-up kit, complete with the medium, techniques, brushes, and paints as the artist, nature, intended them.

2

The Three Pillars of CLEAN7

Ever since I can remember, I wanted to be a doctor. As a kid, when adults asked my friends and me what we wanted to be when we grew up, my friends would go for astronaut, firefighter, inventor, and cowboy. Me, a doctor. I had no doubts. It was already in my blood.

Pillar 1: Functional Medicine

Early on during my time at medical school in Montevideo, Uruguay, I met a remarkable doctor, Roberto Canessa, who would soon become my mentor. He is a traditional cardiologist with a unique story. When he was a teenager, a plane carrying his school rugby team crashed in the Andes mountains and, after an intense but fruitless search, the young men were given up for dead. Of the forty people on board, only sixteen survived. For more than two months, they were stuck inside the fuselage, partially under the snow in freezing temperatures and buried at times after avalanches. In order to survive, they were forced to eat the bodies of their dead friends.

Roberto and another team player, Fernando Parrado, decided not to wait any longer for a rescue team and walked across the mountains in the harshest of conditions until they reached civilization in Chile and told the military about the rest of the survivors and where to find them. When the rescue team arrived and saved the rest of the surviving rugby team, the rescuers could not believe that Roberto and Fernando, despite no equipment and already emaciated from two months of very little food and hardship, had made it to the other side of the mountain. This story is beautifully told in a book called *Alive* and his personal account in his book *I Had to Survive*. Roberto has this incredible life force and a sense that nothing is impossible. When I saw how this affected the way he practiced medicine, I was both inspired and imbued with the same sense that anything is possible and that never left me. He was also the person who talked me into going to New York to study cardiology after I graduated from medical school in 1990.

During my training years at New York University Downtown Hospital and Lenox Hill Hospital in Manhattan, I learned how to apply everything I had learned in medical school to diagnose and treat patients. We were taught to think of the different parts of the body separately and to ask questions that directed us to where the problematic part might be. Symptoms were grouped into syndromes and further into diseases. Laboratory tests were ordered to confirm or rule out the different possible diagnoses, and once confirmed, we were taught which medications to treat the problem with in order to improve the patient's symptoms. Treatment was a matter of either cutting off sick pieces through surgery and reconstructing what was left so that things could work as well as possible or changing the chemistry with medications to make people feel better by attenuating or completely silencing symptoms. The schedule was grueling with long work hours and many overnights on call.

There was no time or reason to question anything. Until I got sick. Really sick. To the point where I couldn't even function. I searched for help and found the best doctors available. The lack of sleep, the stress, the junk food all played a role in my sudden wrestling with depression, allergies, and IBS. Before I knew it, I was on seven different prescription pills and more miserable than ever. This was a pivotal period in my life. For the first time ever, the limits of modern medicine became crystal clear to me. I understood intuitively that what I was experiencing wasn't natural or normal, and I needed help. At the same time, I knew that a lifetime living on medications wasn't going to work. I started to see that I wasn't alone and that there were so many of us suffering from what appeared to be the direct result of simply living in our modern world. I took the skills I had learned as a doctor and decided to look for different solutions.

After graduating as a cardiologist, my first stop was an ashram in India, where I learned meditation, lived a vegetarian lifestyle, tried basic Ayurvedic principles and other healing modalities, and I started to get better. But as soon as I returned to the United States and joined a busy cardiology practice, the symptoms came back with a vengeance.

The jackpot moment was when I found the concepts and practices of detoxification at a spa in Palm Springs, The We Care Spa. I had heard remarkable transformations were occurring there. When I checked it out and experienced it myself, my health issues were completely resolved and I no longer needed any medications. An intense detox program at We Care made me healthy again, even though at the time I did not understand how. The results were undeniable and I became ravenous in my efforts to understand the science of how and why it worked. I spent countless hours at We Care talking to every guest and learning from the owner and founder Susana Belen. Eventually I started lecturing there and guiding people on how to handle their medical issues while detoxing. After Palm Springs I moved to Los Angeles where I joined the Golden Cabinet, an integrative medicine center founded by Dr. Drew Francis, a Chinese medicine practitioner and gifted acupuncturist.

Dr. Francis explained that Chinese medicine also considers the accumulation of toxins as the basis of most chronic diseases and that a relatively new school of medicine would help me make sense of everything from a scientific point of view. This was the school of Functional Medicine, which he had been studying for some time. Dr. Francis insisted that I sign up for a weekend course called AFMCP (Applying Functional Medicine in Clinical Practice). I found out that one such course was being offered close to Los Angeles and signed up. The AFMCP completely changed the course of my medical practice. I met physicians, nutritionists, chiropractors, naturopaths, and many other health care practitioners there as well, all transformed by this three-day course.

Functional Medicine is what Western modern medicine has evolved into as a result of rethinking its knowledge and data from a more natural worldview, looking at systems and functions and the relationship with our environment and social network. Another way of putting this is that Western modern medicine doctors turn into Functional Medicine doctors when they are trained to think like Ayurvedic or Chinese medicine practitioners. The most inspiring lecturer was also the father of Functional Medicine, Jeffrey Bland.

Dr. Bland explained that Functional Medicine represents an operational system that focuses on the underlying causes of disease from a systems biology perspective and that engages the patient and practitioner in a therapeutic partnership. It specifically focuses on detox and the processes that happen in the liver, the intestines, the skin, the lymph nodes, and the kidneys, among others. If you talk to different specialists about each of these processes separately, they will obviously know about them. But most Western allopathic (traditional) medicine doctors will really know about detox only as it relates to the organ or tissue they specialize in, rather than putting everything together as a whole system or group of systems. Even fewer doctors understand about the energetics of detox, the psychological and emotional implications, and how to deal with all these things while guiding a patient through a detox program.

It is difficult to express the feeling I had by the third day of the AFMCP. It was as if I had been blindfolded and someone had just ripped off my blinders. And I wasn't the only one. We all wanted to talk to Jeffrey Bland, who is changing the approach to medical care before our very eyes. I bought the *Textbook of Functional Medicine* and it hasn't left my side ever since.

I dived into Functional Medicine with every bit of my energy. All of my experience and research had led me to this point. Healing patients from a holistic model was empowering and the results were astounding. The more I learned, the more I realized how many people were in need of the healing wisdom of Functional Medicine and the principles and practices of detoxification in particular. I was desperate to share this knowledge with more people. I went to work like a mad scientist putting together what would become my first book, *CLEAN*, and the CLEAN program.

A few days after the release of *CLEAN* I got a phone call from an unknown number. "Hi, Dr. Junger, this is Jeffrey Bland calling," said the voice on the other end. He invited me to Seattle to meet his team in person. I remember being nervous when introducing myself to everyone. Imagine if you just start playing guitar and singing and finally you record a song of your own. Imagine then that Mick Jagger somehow hears your song and invites you for a jam session with the Rolling Stones. That is how I felt when I was with this group of incredible minds. I officially became a Functional Medicine doctor and have been studying and practicing it ever since.

Functional Medicine in CLEAN7

I learned many things from Functional Medicine. It rearranged all my knowledge from medical school and years of working at hospitals. It also helped me understand other healing tools I had found and continue to find. There are two basic Functional Medicine principles that go to the heart of CLEAN7: (a) the Elimination Diet and (b) the Five Rs.

The Elimination Diet

The Elimination Diet is about getting rid of the most common dietary triggers. These are foods that cause or mediate inflammatory reactions, immune irritation, hormonal imbalance, allergic reactions, or anything else that interferes with optimal function in one way or another. It is a primarily plant-based approach that includes organic and unprocessed foods high in antioxidants, vitamins, beneficial phytochemicals, minerals, fiber, and essential fatty acids. It excludes more than four thousand foreign toxic chemicals, xenobiotics, found in food as additives, as well as hormones, antibiotics, saturated and trans fats, sugar, and other empty calories, all of which are an everyday reality for millions of people around the world. The Elimination Diet has become one of my most useful tools to help people with their health issues.

When I meet patients for the first time, it is not always clear where or what to look for to explain their symptoms. Doctors take a medical history, do a physical examination, and send for initial screening lab tests. Once the results come back, if there are abnormalities, it narrows down the possible diagnosis. While I wait for the lab test results, I put most of my patients on the Elimination Diet. By the time their lab tests are back and by their second appointment, more than half my patients' problems have been greatly if not completely resolved. The Elimination Diet takes away the foods that aggravate the body, giving the immune system a much-needed rest and allowing the body's natural healing mechanisms to function properly and resolve the underlying issues.

Many patients come to me after taking food allergy tests. Too often the results of these tests just bring confusion. Many foods to which we are intolerant do not cause an allergic-type reaction mediated by immunoglobulins, which is what most of these tests measure. In turn, many foods can cause an allergic-type reaction that doesn't show up in the test. Such a reaction stays under the radar, without the typical allergic-type symptoms, and adds to the dysfunction in the body. Other foods cause an allergic reaction amplified enough to show symptoms, sometimes dramatically as hives or wheezing, but often the foods that cause them can revert to being nonallergic foods once problems such as "leaky gut" are corrected. I rarely use food allergy tests. Instead, the Elimination Diet is the key tool to understanding food reactions.

In medical terms, a period of time on the Elimination Diet reduces antigenicity and inflammatory reactions, allows repair of gut hyperpermeability, rebalances cytokines, and improves digestion and absorption. After a strict period on the Elimination Diet, you slowly reintroduce the different foods you have avoided, one by one, to detect which ones might be causing disruption. During the Elimination Diet period, it is more important to know what *not* to eat than what *to eat*. As long as you avoid the proscribed foods, you are good. Of course, it is important to learn which foods to eat. For most people, this is a lengthier process. No food allergy test is as accurate or as useful as a period of time on the Elimination Diet, followed by reintroduction of different foods. Since the integrity of your intestinal wall is always changing, some foods can act as trigger foods at times and not at other times. That is why the Elimination Diet is not a one-time test that determines your food sensitivities for life. I recommend going through periods of the Elimination Diet periodically. As time goes by you get to really know yourself and when your sensitivities to different foods change without needing to test them with reintroduction.

The Elimination Diet seems drastic to a lot of people. Suddenly removing dairy, sugar, gluten, alcohol, and coffee (the big five) plus a list of other foods, such as oranges, strawberries, and nightshades (eggplants, tomatoes, peppers) all at once from your diet, is something that many people cannot wrap their minds around. I understand that this is a tough mental hurdle. Eliminating just one of these items alone can sound challenging. Many of my patients try to negotiate. "What if I eat half of the bread I normally eat? Can I use milk only in my tea?" I stay firm and inspire them to do it all at once, cold turkey. What most people find out is that it is easier to drop all these foods at once than one by one. And even better news, the results are amazing. You will be following the Elimination Diet during CLEAN7 as your baseline diet and you will take one step further, by personalizing it according to your Ayurvedic type. (See Find Your Dosha on page 156.)

The Five Rs: Remove, Restore, Repair, Reinoculate, Relax

Remove

The first R calls to *Remove* all foods that cause any kind of negative effect on the body. Eliminating all processed, food-like products loaded with chemicals is paramount. Only whole foods. But even certain whole foods can affect you negatively in many different ways. These ways include acidification (which can lead to diarrhea and osteoporosis), mucus formation (which causes congestion and a runny nose), constipation, immune response (skin issues), inflammation, and a myriad of other expressions of food sensitivities.

It is also important to remove the chemicals from other sources. Go to www.cleanprogram.com/clean7 for links to the best resource on how to eliminate toxins in your home.

Another key aspect is removing the harmful bacteria from the intestines. On the Elimination Diet you will starve the bad bacteria, allowing the good ones to thrive and survive. On CLEAN7, the selective antimicrobial effect of Ayurvedic herbs will accelerate this process.

Restore

As you remove the obstacles that are preventing you from looking and feeling your best, you need to also restore whatever is lacking. Antioxidants are important to buffer the surge of free radicals that occurs initially when the body starts detoxing intensely. Important as well is the presence and availability of the nutrients needed for the biotransformation and detoxification reactions in the liver and elsewhere. The CLEAN7 recipes have been formulated with this R in mind. They will provide the antioxidants, the fiber, and all the other micronutrients needed to detox and repair.

Repair

Your body has an innate ability to heal itself and is constantly trying to repair whatever damage it suffers. There are two main reasons that repair cannot be achieved at times: (1) obstacles such as toxic molecules or trigger foods that interfere with these processes and (2) things such as specific nutrients needed by the repair cells are lacking. When you remove the obstacles and you provide what is lacking, everything falls into place and repair happens seamlessly.

In Functional Medicine, we understand the importance of empowering the body to reach its full healing potential. Repair is a critical component of CLEAN7. The recipes for the CLEAN7 program were specifically designed to provide all the nutrients necessary—such as glutamine, essential fatty acids, zinc, and many others—to aid the body in this process, especially repairing the intestinal lining and reducing gut permeability. The CLEAN7 Ayurvedic herbs will boost repair as well. In seven days, you can get the repair processes activated, strengthened, and supported.

Reinoculate

A wealth of evidence suggests that the good bacteria in our gut, in the right places and in the correct ratios between species, is vital to our well-being. Affecting your weight, your chances of being obese, becoming diabetic, or having your immune system attack your own cells, the bacteria in your gut have far-reaching consequences well beyond where they live in your body. They feed on whatever you feed yourself. When the good bacteria are fueled by a natural, well-balanced diet they thrive and in turn help the body in many ways that we are yet discovering. These good bacteria, however, die when fed highly processed food-like products or any real food with preservatives. These chemicals are put in foods to prevent the bacteria from growing and spoiling it, completely disregarding the fact that they will also spoil your intestinal flora.

The unnatural way in which we eat ends up changing our intestines in a negative way, creating a condition known as dysbiosis. This is a major contributor to hyperpermeability, or leaky gut, which is at the very root of many of today's chronic diseases. The CLEAN7 program will starve the bad bacteria. Ayurvedic herbs will help not only in reducing bad bacteria but also in selectively feeding the good ones, repopulating the intestines with the right bacteria in the optimal ratio. If it's in your reach, using probiotics will accelerate a beneficial bacterial reinoculation.

Relax

Functional Medicine teaches the importance of the mind-body connection. It promotes the use of many tools such as biofeedback, meditation, movement, fun activities, and vacation time. During CLEAN7 use the meditation techniques described in chapter 5. So many people are intimidated by the word *meditation* and their misconception of what it is. The techniques I offer you are simple and short and can be done at any time of the day. And they really help.

Pillar 2: Ayurvedic Medicine

Growing up in Uruguay in a Jewish family, I often heard stories of rabbis who had incredible gifts. My dad used to tell me stories of a legendary rabbi, the Baal Shem Tov, who was believed to understand the language of animals and plants and could heal the sick. My mom is very open-minded, a real equal opportunity saint admirer. She often takes flowers and other offerings to different saints. Her favorite is Saint Expedite who is famous in South America for the resolution of health and all other kinds of problems in people who pray to him. Later, during my years in medical school I studied with Pablo Jourdan, who by our second year also started studying to be a Catholic priest. Half our study time would be spent on medicine, the other half on discussions about religion and spirituality. He told me stories of the healing powers that Jesus had and that he believed when it is said that Jesus could make the blind see, it was not a metaphor, it was literal. He not only believed these healings had happened, but he also believed they did not contradict science, even if they seemed to defy everything that we were studying at the time. He reasoned that a miracle is something that we don't yet have an explanation for. Pablo became a doctor and a priest and today is a bishop in Uruguay and is still a big influence in my life. I have always been a seeker—someone who craves knowledge wherever I can find it. That is one of the reasons I traveled to an ashram in India after graduating as a cardiologist in New York.

When I started working with Ayurvedic doctors at the ashram's first aid station, I immediately started asking questions about the origins and practice of Ayurvedic Medicine. I heard amazing stories of miraculous healings by enlightened beings such as Shirdi Sai Baba, Ramakrishna, Paramahansa Yogananda, Bhagawan Nityananda, Buddha, Ramana Maharshi, and Papaji, to name just a few.

Dr. Manisha, an Ayurvedic doctor volunteering at the ashram's clinic, told me that thousands of years ago the ancient rishis, enlightened yogis also known as seers, translated into words the laws and rules of nature, as they were able to understand its language. This became the blueprint of the whole healing science and system known as Ayurvedic Medicine. For thousands of years, it was transmitted verbally, and its practice was passed down from master to student until it was written down in Sanskrit in ancient scriptures known as the Vedas and the Samhitas, which are the textbooks of Ayurvedic Medicine. The word *Ayurveda* is Sanskrit for *knowledge of life* and it is pretty much an instruction manual for a sophisticated vehicle, meaning the human body, dictated by its designer and manufacturer, namely nature. This "art and science of life" is not only concerned with the individual living machine, your body, but also how it interacts and is interconnected with all of nature and the universe as a whole. According to Ayurveda, nature is the ultimate physician. Inside each living organism is the knowledge not only of how to function but also of how to repair, restore, heal, and even rejuvenate. When a living organism finds itself living in natural conditions, all functions are aligned, there is order and balance and the result is vibrant health. Imbalances occur when the natural order is disrupted. This is why disease begins. The unnatural toxic obstacles (*ama*) must be removed and whatever is lacking must be provided to recreate a more natural inner environment for healing and for successfully carrying on optimal day-to-day body functions.

The history of Ayurvedic Medicine and the stories of amazing healings were fascinating, but they got real, fast, when I witnessed how its practice helped people right there at the ashram's clinic.

Veronica came to the clinic feeling sick. We all sat in a circle as usual, together with Dr. Manisha, Dr. Lee, a Chinese medicine practitioner, and Tom, a nurse who also taught meditation. Veronica had a fever, was vomiting regularly, and had a rash all over her body. The rash was scaring her as it was spreading across her cheeks and forehead. I asked if she had started taking any new medications, as her symptoms could fit with a drug allergic reaction, but she had not. I looked for insect bites, but she had none. Dr. Manisha asked a few questions about her personality and her eating and sleeping habits and how she responded to stress in her life. Veronica was slender, with reddish hair and freckles. She described herself as passionate, with a bit of a temper. She had regular sleeping habits but had been waking up with vivid dreams. She had arrived at the ashram during the hot season from Australia and had been thirsty and sweating profusely from the moment she landed. She had been drinking lots of water, and her favorite, mango juice, all day long. After we all finished asking and examining, we each gave our opinion and our recommendations. I was convinced Veronica was having a bad allergic reaction and wanted to start her on antihistamines right away and possibly corticosteroids if her rash worsened or her breathing became difficult.

Dr. Manisha had a completely different take. She said Veronica had a Pitta constitution (predominant fire-water dosha) and the fire element in her was out of control. She recommended that Veronica stop drinking mango juice since it was a very heating food, as well as to avoid all spicy foods, keep as cool as she could, and stay out of the sun. She also prescribed her a combination of herbs. Dr. Manisha argued that antihistamines and corticosteroids would just mask the symptoms but agreed that they would be necessary if things did not improve. Veronica decided to follow the Ayurvedic advice. A few days later her skin went back to normal and all other symptoms disappeared. She also reported that her meditation practice had greatly improved and she was sleeping better.

Ayurvedic Medicine could not always give the best solution to our patients. There are acute problems that are better dealt with by modern medicine. For example, one day, one of the monks came to the clinic with shortness of breath. His ankles were mildly swollen. He was overweight and had been a smoker in his "previous life" as a stockbroker. He did not have chest pain or any other symptoms.

He did not even want to hear the Western medical advice, so we skipped my evaluation and went directly to Dr. Manisha's. After dietary advice and an emphatic order to rest, the monk got up and left. I had a strong feeling that he needed an electrocardiogram so I ran after him and convinced him to let me do one back at the clinic. It showed that he had suffered a heart attack in the past, or more than one. After a long talk I managed to get him in a car and drive him to a modern hospital in Mumbai. The chief cardiologist there agreed with me that his mild shortness of breath was probably indicating a bigger problem than it seemed. His legs were swollen with edema. The cardiologist did an angiogram that day and found that there was a 99 percent blockage of the mid left anterior descending (LAD) coronary artery, which was feeding the only part of his heart that had not been affected by at least two heart attacks. The local cardiologist wanted to send him for bypass surgery, but the monk refused. Instead, he had a stent put in, which saved his life. Once he was back at the ashram he followed Dr. Manisha's advice to a T, but I had to police him to ensure that he took his aspirin and other heart meds. I heard he did well for many years after that. Ayurvedic Medicine helped once the emergency situation was taken care of. There is nothing better than modern Western medicine for acute problems such as strokes, heart attacks, and broken bones. The problem is that modern medicine uses the same tools for chronic problems, and they just don't work.

Time after time I witnessed the ashram's Ayurvedic doctors tackle a wide range of illnesses. My first experiences with Ayurvedic Medicine convinced me of the profound benefits of this ancient healing system. When I returned to the United States and started practicing cardiology in Palm Springs, I was hoping to find Ayurvedic Medicine doctors that I could work with. Unfortunately, I quickly became too busy to even think about it, and I barely had time to see all the patients assigned to me.

While I was not actively studying or learning more, I couldn't shake what I had learned about Ayurveda. Soon after moving to Palm Springs to work as a cardiologist, I stumbled upon the concepts and practices of detoxification. As I mentioned in the previous chapter, a detox program completely restored my health and I became obsessed with understanding how. Many books I found had isolated principles from Ayurveda but it was Functional Medicine that gave me the answers I was looking for. Ayurvedic Medicine was still a little bit of a mystery to me until a few years later.

Functional Medicine gave me the tools to start a worldwide movement with my first book, *CLEAN*, and the CLEAN program. And *CLEAN* ultimately took me back to India to sit with and witness an Ayurvedic Medicine master in action who cleared up any confusion I had about it. In chapter 6, I will tell you in detail how I met Dr. Narendra Singh. He was the one who completely demystified that ancient science and taught me how to apply general Ayurvedic principles and tools to my practice.

Dr. Narendra was also a Western medicine physician, so he spoke the scientific language. He said I already had an Ayurvedic mindset. The fact that I was focusing on detoxification as a powerful tool in my medical practice proved it. Ayurvedic Medicine pays special attention to detoxification. He explained that the Sanskrit word *ama* refers to the toxic load and Ayurveda considers its elimination the necessary first step in any healing plan. Functional Medicine allowed me to understand how many of the Ayurvedic principles actually worked from a molecular biological point of view.

One of my goals with CLEAN7 is to demystify Ayurveda. Below is a brief overview that will be instrumental in your overall understanding of how your body functions.

Ama

The accumulation of endogenous and exogenous (internal and external) toxins and the mucus and fat that the body generates and retains in order to defend itself from them, is collectively called *ama*. Its accumulation is thought to be at the root of most chronic diseases, and many acute ones as well. Ama's properties are cold, wet, heavy, cloudy, malodorous, and impure. Ama also refers to toxic mental and emotional expressions. Toxic thoughts and toxic emotions are a sign of excess of ama and in turn promote its accumulation in the body. Ayurveda places a great emphasis in triggering, enhancing, supporting, and unblocking the detoxification systems in the body and promoting the elimination of ama. Dr. Narendra explained that in addition to considering how to nutritionally support the biotransformation and detoxification reactions, as well as promote the open flow of the elimination channels in the skin, airways, kidneys, and intestines, Ayurveda pays attention to increasing agni, the digestive fire.

Agni

Agni means fire in Sanskrit. Ayurveda understands it as the intelligent light that sparks and powers life. Agni is hot, dry, light, clear, fragrant, and pure. Ayurveda distinguishes between many different subtypes of agni and the bodily functions that each subtype is involved in. Vibrant health depends on the strength and balance of agni in the body. Improper food, emotional disturbances, and even damp or rainy weather can reduce the strength of agni. The type and combinations of food can negatively affect Agni, but excessive amounts of food and the frequency of meals that we are used to, also contribute to its imbalance. Have you ever started a fire and then added too much wood? It suffocates the fire and can even put it out. The constant state of feeding and digesting, typical of our modern lifestyle, similarly weakens and decreases the agni, allowing ama to accumulate. This is one of the reasons intermittent fasting is a core part of CLEAN7. It provides oxygen to your fire as opposed to piling too much wood on top of it.

Watching Dr. Narendra treat patients reminded me of the great results that I had seen at the ashram almost ten years earlier. Dr. Narendra explained that without being an Ayurvedic doctor, I could start using two important Ayurvedic Medicine principles for promoting, strengthening, and supporting detoxification: observing the doshas and using Ayurvedic herbs.

The Doshas

According to Ayurvedic thinking, the five elements—fire, water, air, earth, and ether—are the fundamental bricks with which nature builds everything. The different substances in nature contain all of the elements in different proportions, with usually one or two that predominate. All animals and plants are in turn made of different combinations of the different substances and elements, and these combinations determine how the organisms function and how they respond to inside and outside changes.

The three main ways in which the elements combine to form the different body types, the doshas, or Ayurvedic constitutions are: pitta (predominance of fire and water), kapha (predominance of earth and water), and vata (predominance of ether and air). All three doshas are present in everyone but when you are conceived, you are programmed with an ideal combination in which one of the doshas will predominate. If maintained in balance, that blueprint will ensure vibrant health throughout your life. In Ayurveda this is called your prakriti. This always stays the same and becomes your home base. When you are feeling well, it is because the three different doshas are in balance with the predominant one in check. This is your state of vibrancy as nature designed it to be, your natural state. It means that your diet, your lifestyle, and your environment are affecting your doshas in a healthy way. Most commonly people have a single dominant dosha. They are either pitta, kapha, or vata dominant body type. But in other cases two doshas are dominant over a third—vata-pitta, pitta-kapha and kapha-vata—and even cases in which all three doshas are in equal proportions, called tridoshic.

But as you age and experience circumstantial, environmental, and dietary habit shifts, one or another dosha may throw you out of balance. It is usually the dominant dosha that goes out of balance, but not always. If you are a vata body type, it will be vata-aggravating foods or activities that most commonly throw your predominant vata out of balance, but your pitta may do that on occasion, or your kapha, as well. Determining which dosha is most out of balance governs what you need to do to rebalance your doshas to get back to your home base. Your momentary dosha imbalance is called vikriti.

In other words, when your prakriti (your dosha body type) is in balance, continuing the lifestyle and dietary guidelines for that dosha will keep you well. Consider it your baseline. If you are a pitta, keeping the baseline fire balance is key. You do so by avoiding pitta-aggravating foods and pitta-aggravating habits and in turn engaging in pitta-soothing activities and eating pitta-soothing foods. But if at any given time pitta people have their vata out of whack, avoiding vata-aggravating foods will help them return to baseline, at which time they would revert to following pitta-guiding principles. The pitta person with a "vata attack" (the vikriti at that time) resolves it by soothing the vata, and once it is balanced, goes back to soothing the pitta. This happens to different degrees throughout life.

Knowing which foods to avoid according to your current state of balance or imbalance will enhance detoxification and repair, as well as balance your mood and calm your mind. In general, dosha imbalances negatively affect the digestive fire (*agni*) and promote the buildup of toxins and mucus as well as the fat that the body generates to buffer the irritation (*ama*). This ama circulates throughout the body in the blood stream, clogging the channels, and gets stuck within the tissues, especially fat. According to Ayurveda, every so-called disease is a crisis of *ama* toxicity, due to the aggravated doshas and a weak *agni*. *Ama* is the basic internal root cause of all disease and the doshas play a major role in its accumulation and elimination.

The Doshas in CLEAN7

During CLEAN7 you will use the dosha system in a simplified way, primarily just focusing on avoiding as many of the foods that your current dosha imbalance guidelines recommend. For example, if your predominant dosha imbalance right now (your vikriti) is pitta, you will benefit by avoiding the foods that are "heating." Avoiding just one of these, such as mango, will be beneficial. Avoiding mango and spicy foods will be even better, and so on. As it relates to detoxification, combining the Elimination Diet and the dosha-guided foods to avoid will be both more powerful and more personalized than either one alone. Unlike the Elimination Diet, which must be strictly followed throughout CLEAN7, the dosha aspect is less strict for the purposes of CLEAN7. If you feel too restricted during the program, consuming a few items from your dosha list of foods to avoid is not a crime. There is a balance between doing it 100 percent and not being able to do it at all, and this is one of the rules that you can bend. (More on this in chapter 3.)

The beauty of Ayurveda is that it lives with you and helps you adapt to changes. Knowing your prakriti allows you to navigate for most of your life, and every now and then, when things get out of balance, you find out what your vikriti is to help you get back to balance. (In chapter 3 you will be asked to fill in a questionnaire twice. The first time you answer the questions you will guide your answers by what has been most constant throughout your lifetime; the second time your answer will reflect how you've been feeling the last month or two. The first set of answers will reveal your prakriti, the second set, your vikriti). Even though a trained Ayurvedic doctor can determine your exact dosha combinations and predominance, your prakriti, and your present vikriti by asking questions, looking at your tongue, and feeling your pulse, a basic and well-formulated questionnaire (page 156) is perfectly adequate in the context of doing the CLEAN7 program.

The dosha system is much more sophisticated and comprehensive than the way that I am using it in CLEAN7. I am focusing on detoxification and borrowing just one aspect from that system. If you resonate with the dosha system and everything else about Ayurveda, you will find that there are many more aspects of balancing your dosha than just avoiding certain foods. Many other aspects of your lifestyle can be modified to promote dosha rebalancing, and different herbs can help too. You may decide to dive deeper into Ayurveda during and after the program. Go to www .cleanprogram.com/clean7 to learn about more ways to benefit from determining your dosha.

Modern and Ancient Medicines Meet

When I started learning about the dosha-related dietary indications, I wondered if its claims were really true. Whenever anyone makes better choices in their diet, they usually see results. Does the dosha consideration truly make a difference? On one of my trips to India I met a remarkable doctor, Shikha Sharma. She is somewhat of a celebrity in India, well known for her books and helping thousands of people across the country with a team of more than one hundred Ayurvedic doctors and nutritionists. I told her about my doubts, and the following was her response.

I can relate to your skepticism. Like you, I was trained in modern medicine at The Maulana Azad Medical College in New Delhi, considered among the top three schools in New Delhi and the top five in India. Naturally I was wary and a tad cynical of this ancient Ayurveda stuff. I didn't even know that in India we have professional colleges offering a five-year degree course in Ayurveda. My curiosity about Ayurveda was sparked when I set up my private practice, a lifestyle disorder and weight management clinic, and I started drawing a blank on questions regarding nutrition for health. I had little knowledge of how to use nutrition to heal the body despite having a medical degree!

Since I had already stepped out of my comfort zone as an allopath, I started reading about Indian Vedic nutrition. A lot of my patients seemed to already know some bits from this ancient knowledge (passed down by their grandmothers). As I started learning Ayurvedic principles of nutrition, health, disease prevention, and its practices, I was mesmerized and humbled by the depth and the logic of this science. I realized that I just had to include the practice of Ayurvedic healing in my practice. To be fair and professional, I hired professional Ayurvedic doctors and nutritionists, so the advice is given directly by them.

Let me give you some examples of how Ayurveda helps our patients:

1. We get obese patients whose weight gets stuck when following the standard weight loss advice, but once we diagnose their prakriti as kapha (water), we stop their consumption of curd and yogurt at night. The resulting decrease in kapha helps them to continue losing weight.

2. The results are also amazing with patients who have a weak liver and a sluggish metabolism. All these cases we start on herbs to detoxify the liver plus dosha-related dietary guidelines. Not only do all the people who are stuck finally move toward weight loss, but they also see an improvement in their skin, energy level, and cholesterol levels.

3. We noticed that women who come to us for weight loss and who have additional problems such as polycystic ovarian syndrome (a metabolic disorder) see a wonderful improvement in metabolic parameters in addition to improving their weight once they start following their dosha diet.

All these cases humbled me as a doctor. We may have made much scientific progress, yet one cannot help but admire the wisdom of the ancients who understood the interconnectedness of nature and humankind.

Ayurvedic Herbs

Nature has endowed plants with incredible abilities. A tangible way to understand this is to think of the unique ability that plants have to produce oxygen through photosynthesis, basically transforming the energetic power of the sun into something that allows life on earth through its spark, when it is used in the body to burn sugar into ATP (adenosine triphosphate). Oxygen carries the fire of the sun into your very cells in a beneficial way that doesn't burn your whole body.

Plants—herbs in particular—have many medicinal qualities.

Herbal medicine is one of the most ancient forms of health care known to humankind. The use of plants for medicinal purposes has been prevalent in many cultures around the world since ancient times and still plays a major role today, even in modern Western medicine. A large percentage of the world's population continues to depend on plants for its basic health care needs, particularly in India and China. Their traditional systems of medicine, Ayurveda and Chinese medicine, are not the only ones that have long used herbal medicines. Tibetan medicine, Greco-Arabic medicine, eclectic medicine, and Japanese Traditional Medicine, known as Kampo, have also used herbs for ages with impressive success. This is also true in Africa, South America, and Australia. In Europe, particularly in Germany, plant medicines, phytomedicines, are prescribed just as any other modern medication is. Around 25 percent of modern medications contain at least one ingredient derived from plants.

In Ayurvedic Medicine, the majority of a pharmacy is made up of plants, as food and herbs. There is actually no clear-cut distinction between the two, as many herbs are consumed as foods, and plant-based foods work in the same way as herbs to promote healing. Both provide nutrients, antioxidants, minerals, and other beneficial molecules and both can affect the body energetically. It was easy for me to understand the first part as I had learned quite a bit about the nutrient part of herbs, but the concept of their energetics took me a little longer to grasp.

When Dr. Narendra spoke about the mechanism of action of herbs, he referred to their prana. "What is prana?' I asked. "It is the life force within every living being. The prana of plants is pure. If it's not altered by humans, the intelligence of plants—its consciousness—is intact, completely aligned with nature, and by resonance can affect our prana. The prana of herbs can restore any distortion that our prana is affected by, therefore restoring the inner self-healing ability."

Dr. Narendra loved certain herbs for detoxification more than others, and his results with patients are legendary, not only in India but also across the world. The ancient Ayurvedic texts describe not only what herbs are useful for what, and why, but also how to grow or obtain them in the wild. His favorite herbs for a detox program are tulsi, turmeric, ashwagandha, moringa, brahmi, and triphala. He always put his female patients on shatavari as well. For the CLEAN7 program I have chosen Dr. Narendra's favorite herbs for detox. It is not mandatory to take all of them during the program. You will get results even without herbs, but they will enhance everything. Using one is better than none. Using two is better than one. And so on.

(See chapters 3 and 4 for details and visit www.cleanprogram.com/clean7 to learn about each of these herbs.)

Pillar 3: Intermittent Fasting

One of my most vivid early childhood memories is of my whole family fasting (or attempting to) on Yom Kippur, the Jewish Day of Atonement. It was strange to have a day in which we didn't eat from the moment the first star came up one evening until the first star appeared on the next. Then we would all get together, usually at my aunt Selma's house, for a ceremony to break the fast with lots of wonderful Jewish delicacies. Before feasting we would hear the stories about why Jews fast on Yom Kippur. After a few years of being unable to complete the fast, I finally did it successfully during Yom Kippur for two consecutive years. At school, my Catholic friends would fast for Lent. Pablo, my study partner in medical school, told me that Jesus Christ, before the most intense part of his life, fasted for forty days and forty nights. I always put fasting on the religious bookshelf in my inner library. It wasn't unfamiliar to me, but we weren't that religious, so I never got into it. Once I left my parent's home, it became just a memory of family life.

As an adult, when I became interested in Eastern spirituality and Eastern spiritual teachers, I started to learn that many more people used fasting for spiritual purposes, including Hindus, Muslims, and Buddhists and I read about its benefits from a yogic, spiritual point of view. Every spiritual master used fasting as a way of advancing spiritually. Furthermore, fasting was used by Gandhi and others as a form of peaceful protest. It was all very interesting, but as a doctor, I didn't link fasting with physical health.

Fasting for health and an awareness of the different types of fasting practices didn't really come alive for me until I first went to the We Care Spa in Desert Hot Springs. There I started learning about fasting as it relates to cleansing and detoxification. I read as many books about fasting as I could get my hands on and experimented with different forms of fasting. One of the first books I read was Arnold Ehret's *Mucusless Diet Healing System.* Another really good book is *Fasting and Eating for Health* by Dr. Joel Fuhrman. It became clear to me that fasting in different forms is beneficial for the body and for overall good health. The verb *fast* is of Germanic origin (*fasten*). Fasting plays a more significant and mainstream medical role in Germany, where many hospitals even have wings dedicated to people who do long fasts. It is also widely used in Russia. Fasting not only has ancient roots, it is currently being used around the world as a necessary healing tool.

The Laws of Nature

One of the best explanations I found for why fasting is so clearly beneficial is the concept of further realignment of our gene activity with nature. Animals in the wild live in a way that imposes upon them an ongoing cycle of feasting followed by fasting. They feast when they find food and then they fast until they find the next meal. In general, plant-eating species have the least difficulty in finding the next meal. Meat eaters, on the other hand, which must find prey to kill, have feasting-fasting cycles with longer fasts. Nature's design for animals is intermittent feasting and fasting. From the beginning of our evolution and for hundreds of thousands of years, our ancestors lived similarly to other animals, alternating between feasting and fasting. Our genes evolved in this way and they work best directing the body's metabolism the closer they get to these conditions.

Store or Die

Obtaining calories for energy and building blocks to make our bodies and enable them to function depends completely on food, so life depends on food. Over thousands of years the human body evolved and adapted in a way that prioritizes the best use of food once it crosses your lips. As a result, whenever food was found and consumed, the body prioritized digestion, and other processes would slow down or even shut off so as to not interfere with digestion. Our genes evolved in a way that shifts physiology and behavior so that food can be properly digested, absorbed, assimilated, and any excess stored. After a big meal, animals slow down. Many even fall asleep, a way to avoid their muscles using up the precious energy needed to process the meal.

Have you noticed that after huge meals you get tired and fall asleep? You may have even heard of the scientific explanation that there is an alkaline tide or wave in your blood stream, the result of acid being poured into the stomach, which makes you fall asleep. That is just the biochemical description of what nature put in place to do exactly what is discussed above, slow you down. There are other hormonal changes that are triggered after a meal. The most obvious example is a surge in insulin, but it is not the only one. These hormonal and behavioral shifts create the conditions for the body to absorb as much food as possible and store as much as possible as well. The body enters into a digestion-absorption-storage mode and the brain around the intestines kind of takes over even putting the other brain (in the skull) to sleep. I'll call it the "feasting state" for simplicity. In the feasting state you become sleepy, your thinking slows down, your ambition to do anything else gets reduced, and your fat cells grow as they store everything that is not needed at that moment. Other processes in the body also slow down to allow most of the energy that they would be consuming to be diverted to the life-preserving act of handling food. One of these groups of processes are the processes of detoxification and elimination. They get reduced to the minimum necessary. The body knows it is supposed to catch up later when all the work of digestion and absorption is done. This is all by nature's incredibly intelligent design and centuries of gene adaptation.

After a good post-feasting rest, life continues. The daily activities begin: walking, thinking, working. Digestion, absorption, and storage are completed and you become more awake and alert. In natural conditions, as time goes by and no food is eaten, the "feasting state" winds down. Slowly, hunger sets in, changing behavior. A sense of energy and alertness arises, which will be necessary to find or hunt the next meal. This is the beginning of the "fasting state," the other side of the coin, both absolutely necessary for optimal health because of our genetic evolution. The storage-promoting hormones disappear and other hormones surge to promote the utilization of stored energy, minerals, vitamins, proteins, etc.

Now the body starts tapping into fat stores and burning them for energy. To do this, fat must first be converted into ketone bodies, creating a state of ketosis, which happens concomitantly with everything else that is happening in the fasting state. Some of the benefits of ketosis may result from the presence of ketone bodies, and some just because the process of digesting food is not using up most of the body's energy. When ketosis results from eating certain foods (which is what a keto diet is designed to achieve), the benefits are less than when ketosis happens as part of the fasting state. During this state other important processes are also promoted physiologically and behaviorally. More energy is now allotted to the detoxification processes, plus the recently absorbed nutrients needed for optimal function will be available, making these processes more likely to be completed successfully. Healing and repairing processes get a better chance as well. When animals are unwell, their natural instinct is to rest and abstain from eating. You may have observed this with your cat or dog. When people are sick they lose their appetite. The body demands rest in order to heal and may even impose it. Nature, the physician within, knows what's best. If enough time passes without eating, energy stores will be depleted and the body will start eating itself, a state called autophagia. Many believe that the body will start consuming the least necessary cells first, especially the diseased ones. This may explain some of the countless and seemingly miraculous stories about the healing power of fasting.

Evolution Confusion, Stone Age Bodies in a Fast-Food World

Imagine waking up one day and the sun never sets again. Only day, no night, forever. What would happen to life as you know it? Or just eternal winter without summer. It is unthinkable. It would be unsustainable. For our genes, after eons of optimally evolving with nature by feasting and fasting, suddenly being only in the feasting state without intermittent episodes of being in the fasting state is as if you were kept awake indefinitely. Confusion would soon set in and all kinds of problems would begin. Part of nature's way of functioning is that genes take thousands of years to evolve. Natural conditions are pretty constant over time and genes have the necessary time to evolve slowly and steadily. For centuries humans had no way of storing food in order to eat at a later time. In a timeline that represents the period in which we have been evolving on the planet, the years in which we had food available 24/7/365 is a microscopic dot. The supermarkets we take for granted, where most humans buy their food today, are not even that old. King Kullen, the world's first supermarket, opened its doors in New York City in 1930. Our genes have not even had time to detect this new constant feasting state as a push to evolve and even less to make the necessary evolutionary changes. Our genes are busy directing the body to do what it took so long to learn: when food is present, slow everything else down, so it can be digested, absorbed, assimilated, and stored, as if this is the last meal for a while. There's no way the genes can know that two hours from now you're going to eat more food. By doing so, you are keeping your body only in the state of feasting and never allowing it to go into the fasting state, ever. Most people living in the modern industrialized world have never been in the state of fasting.

We are now aware of how eating unnatural foods can decimate your health. We also understand how eating too much and too often can do the same, even when eating only natural foods. The way I see it is this is not nature's punishment for gluttony. It is just a preservation-survival safety feature in Nature's design. The planet would not survive if for some reason one of its species started eating everything in sight. So it included a self-sickening mechanism within its design.

Even if you eat the healthiest, whole, organic, in-season foods, it is just not natural to do it all the time. Think of feasting and fasting as polar states, the up and down, the on and off, the yin and yang, the balance of which is essential for well-being. The constant state of feasting is killing us, making us obese, and creating the conditions for disease to set in. Constant feasting weakens agni, impairs detoxification, blocks healing and repairing, reduces agility, and even dampens mental clarity. What happened? How did we get here?

Breakfast, Lunch, and Dinner—Says Who?

Having three meals a day is something that humans have been doing only relatively recently in an evolutionary time frame. Food historians suggest that among the sea of changes initiated by the industrial revolution was a significant change in eating patterns. Once people started working outside the home and on the company's clock, they began to eat their midday meal, which had traditionally been what we now call dinner, at or near their workplace. The evening meal, which had been formerly something light such as tea and toast, became the large meal it is today. The idea of breakfast, lunch, and dinner evolved because of a cultural, societal need for comfort and practicality. This shift in behavior quickly became a commercial enterprise and entire industries were born. Breakfast, lunch, and dinner set the day's rhythm.

Meals are an integral part of life. We talk and share with our family during dinner. We wish each other a good day during breakfast and help each other organize the day. We cook for the ones we love. We celebrate with meals around a table. Parties revolve around meals. Our day is divided around meal times. Our work schedule is marked by meals. We pay a lot of attention to planning where and what to eat next. Some of us suffer anxiety around meals if we are health conscious and nothing healthy is available. We get cranky when we get past mealtime without eating. At some point we stop whatever else we are doing, as important as it may be, to have a meal. Life revolves around meals. Nobody questions it. Breakfast, lunch, and dinner are the way things are. You sleep, you wake up, you have breakfast, you go to school or work, you have lunch, you keep working, you have dinner, you go back to sleep. This is life. Or is it? Three meals a day, and snacking in between them, is as unnatural as the sea of toxins in which we are swimming. And it's driving our genes crazy. I don't see this cultural habit changing anytime soon. But I do see many people rewriting their own script by skipping meals and shifting the frequency with which they eat and making it fit into a regular social life. You can easily fit intermittent fasting into your lifestyle, no matter what it is.

What Is Intermittent Fasting?

Fasting is voluntarily electing not to eat beyond the time when we would normally be having our next meal and for a determined period of time after that. Intermittent fasting is doing that intermittently, alternating periods when we eat as we always do with periods of fasting. During the time we don't eat we drink only water and/or herbal teas, but nothing with any caloric value. The whole use of language around fasting is very confusing. There is no single definition when we refer to fasting, nor is there a single set of rules. How many hours of not eating does it take to be considered fasting?

Are we all fasting at night while sleeping? Is breakfast how we all break our daily fast?

A useful way to think about fasting is as it relates to what happens in your body. Approximately eight hours after your last meal, depending on how big it was, your body completes the process of digesting, absorbing, and assimilating it. This is when the body refocuses from digestion to other vital matters such as detoxification. Detoxification doesn't stop while digestion is taking place; it is simply slowed down, just as thinking and moving are. If we eat again as soon as the body finishes digesting, we bounce back into the feasting mode. Eight hours is not enough time for the body to even enter into the fasting mode, which takes approximately twelve hours to begin to set in. So, in terms of fasting, a window of twelve hours between the last meal of one day and the first meal of the next is the minimum required to give your detox processes the time and energy to catch up with the necessary work of maintaining inner cleanliness.

Nobody can specify exactly the timing of the physiologic changes that occur after twelve hours—it is different for everyone. Gradually the gut starts to feel empty, a sensation that is deeply satisfying. The mind starts to clear and there is a surge of energy. Physiologically, the body shifts into obtaining energy from stored reserves, which eventually is mostly from fat. Although glucose stored in the liver and muscles as glycogen is initially burned, ketone bodies start eventually appearing in the blood and are used as fuel. Detoxification intensifies and repair accelerates. The more hours you allow your body to experience this state, the more intense the benefits you will reap. By the time twenty-four hours have elapsed these beneficial changes reach a great level of intensity.

To Fast or Not to Fast . . .

It is mind-blowing that as a society we have disrupted our natural rhythms so much so that we have all but eliminated the body's best chances of being in a state of balance. Many of us have never been in the fasting state for a single hour in our lives. If not practiced for religious purposes, fasting remains an "alternative" treatment and is not considered beneficial by conventional medicine. Furthermore, there are lots of misunderstandings about it, which make fasting a taboo for many. Whether these reasons are generated and fueled by simple misunderstandings, or intentionally by the powers that be, to maintain the status quo of constantly being fed, I will leave up to you to decide.

A common reason for many people to discard the idea of fasting at all is that they label themselves as hypoglycemic. It is true that some people may fall into hypoglycemia as a result of real and serious medical problems, such as when certain glands don't function properly. It may happen by mistake in the management of certain medical conditions, such as diabetes, when someone self-administers too much insulin. A diabetic who uses too much insulin may go into hypoglycemia. But most of the people I encounter who are concerned about being hypoglycemic are talking only about the way they feel when they don't eat for a while. I understand that it can be uncomfortable but it is not a medical issue and what they are experiencing is due mostly to conditioning of their body. This feeling is the body demanding a sugar or stimulant high, in whatever form it can get it. The good news is that it doesn't take long to train your body to not respond in this way.

Another common reason for shunning fasting is the belief that it will slow your metabolism and make you gain weight. The logic is that by lowering caloric intake we are training the body to eat less and store more and that over time this will affect the number of calories we can consume without gaining weight. This thinking is also behind the common advice by nutritionists and personal trainers to eat six smaller meals a day. There is some truth to the fact that digestion takes energy and therefore burns calories. But this is not what defines our metabolic rate. Your muscle mass determines that.

The fear of losing muscle mass is another common reason from abstaining from fasting. Studies have shown that this is not the case during intermittent fasting schedules. Intermittently entering the fasting state has been proven beneficial for weight loss. I once met the actor Hugh Jackman who told me that he used intermittent fasting together with exercise and proper nutrition to get into shape for *Wolverine*. You have only to look at the shape he was in to see that he broke all these myths. Some people equate fasting with starving, which has negative medical and cultural connotations. I understand starving as the state in which the body has no more reserves: and is lacking nutrients to continue bodily functions normally. This is simply not what is happening when intermittently fasting. (See chapter 7 for ways to fast intermittently.)

Fasting the CLEAN7 Way

For all the above reasons, I introduced fasting as one of the pillars of CLEAN7. By gradually increasing the window of time between the last meal of the day and the first meal of the next during the first three days of the program, we are training the body to start entering the fasting state and letting it sit for longer each day. On day 4 your body will be ready to dive into the fasting state more fully, and that is exactly what you will do by fasting for twenty-four hours. By the time you break the fast on day 5 with a liquid meal (smoothie or shake), you will have put your body in the fasting state and basked in it for some time. This potentiates everything that we are trying to achieve by doing CLEAN7. Detoxification intensifies to a level within twenty-four hours that otherwise would take several days to achieve. Your body enters into a state of maximum healing and repair. CLEAN7 is the perfect way to have your first experience of fasting. It prepares your body for three days before fasting to make certain the experience is healing and rejuvenating. It is also the perfect way to introduce fasting into your life for the long run.

When you enter the fasting state, you are creating the conditions necessary for your genes to rest from activating the damage control and unnecessary over-storage. Your genes will recognize this state and instead will be able to activate other activities more intensely. For your genes it will be like having a good night's sleep after a year of sleep deprivation. Your gut will start flattening down in a way and with a speed that you've never experienced before. You will also experience the freedom of not having to plan your next meal. You will be momentarily released from the anxiety that this entails. You will have more time and more energy to do other things. The cells of your intestinal wall will be able to begin to repair themselves faster, or even for the first time in a while. Your sleep will reach new depths. Your puffiness will dramatically reduce. If you have dimples, you will notice them more sharply. Eventually you may see dimples you didn't even know you had, or that you haven't seen since you were a teenager. Things happen when intermittently entering and staying in the fasting state for a few hours that won't happen in any other way, even if you do a detox plan for a full year. You have to experience it. This is the fuel injection for the CLEAN7 engine.

The three pillars of CLEAN7—Functional Medicine, Ayurvedic Medicine, and intermittent fasting—complement and potentiate each other. This is why in seven days you will be able to see results that would otherwise take you much longer to achieve. It took me decades of study, research, and trials to find the information and practices that I have packed in to *CLEAN7*. You will get them in seven days, and they will last you a lifetime.

3

Getting Ready for CLEAN7

You are about to start CLEAN7, a week-long detox program based on principles from Functional Medicine, Ayurvedic Medicine, and intermittent fasting. In practical terms, Functional Medicine will have you avoiding certain foods according to the Elimination Diet, which includes all those foods most likely to trigger sensitivities, such as milk, gluten, and nightshade vegetables, as well as any food-like products loaded with toxic chemicals. You'll replace the toxic and trigger foods with nutrient-rich whole foods (see Foods to Enjoy on page 154). Ayurvedic Medicine will further personalize your diet according to your dosha constitution and will help support the detox process through the use of herbs in supplemental form. Following CLEAN7's protocol for mealtimes will result in intermittent fasting. You will start with about twelve hours between dinner and breakfast the following day, working up to a twenty-four-hour fast, while drinking plenty of herbal tea and water.

Is CLEAN7 for You?

If you are pregnant or breastfeeding, it is not a time to engage in any detox program. This is a time to rest and nurture your baby and yourself. Also, if you have any advanced disease that requires medications and medical care, do this program only under direct supervision from your physician. Medications that need consistent blood levels may be more or less absorbed with any drastic change in diet, which can lead to changes in blood levels. Anti-arrhythmic, antiepileptics, anticoagulants, hormones, and chemotherapy agents are examples of the medications that can be affected by a detox program. Type 1 diabetics should attempt any such program only under close supervision by someone with experience with it. If you fall into any of these categories, please consult your doctor before attempting to do CLEAN7, or better yet, find a Functional Medicine practitioner in your area (you can search by Zip code at https://www.ifm.org/find-a-practitioner/).

To successfully do the CLEAN7 program, you will need certain materials and ingredients, make certain preparations, and get your head in the right place. If you feel especially toxic, or even if not but you want a smoother transition, you can prep with a pre-cleanse. Let's look at these steps one by one.

Set Your Intention and Turn It on Fire

There is nothing as powerful as the desire to set your intention on fire. When you truly desire something, you will make it happen and let nothing get in your way. Think about the other things you have really desired in your life, whether being with a certain person, having a child, achieving certain career goals, or even owning a particular pair of fabulous shoes. Chances are you have achieved those things. Even if you feel unsure about how or whether to pursue the desired person, thing, or state of being, you leap over hurdles to achieve what you desire. In this case, there is nothing to be unsure about: the instructions are easy to follow. What you need to bring is your commitment, and it will be stronger the more you desire it. You can fuel your desire for something if you visualize what it can do for you:

- Envision a different you. Close your eyes and picture your life today. How do you look on a typical day? How do you feel?

- What would it mean to look and feel younger and to have more energy and enthusiasm for life? How might that feel?

- How would your family and close friends feel if the health issues that limit you disappeared?

- How would it benefit you in social, financial, spiritual, and emotional terms to live in a state of vibrant energy and mental clarity?

Visualize these possibilities in detail; sense what they feel like. Notice how the spark of desire ignites a wildfire when you begin to feel the possibility of change. Set your intention to commit to the program from day 1 and complete it. Keep a strong vision of the positive changes that doing CLEAN7 will bring to your life.

Print Out the CLEAN7 Protocol

Making sure you have the seven-day protocol at your fingertips at all times. Print out a copy of the image below, snap a photo of it on your cell phone, or make a paper copy to post on your fridge or bulletin board. That way, whether you're at home or away, you will never be without it.

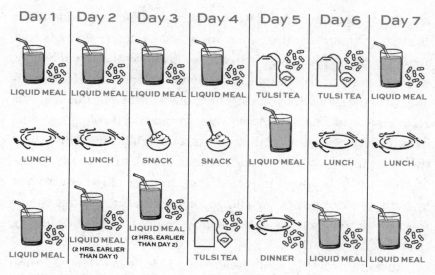

Day 1	Day 2	Day 3	Day 4	Day 5	Day 6	Day 7
LIQUID MEAL	LIQUID MEAL	LIQUID MEAL	LIQUID MEAL	TULSI TEA	TULSI TEA	LIQUID MEAL
LUNCH	LUNCH	SNACK	SNACK	LIQUID MEAL	LUNCH	LUNCH
LIQUID MEAL	LIQUID MEAL (2 HRS. EARLIER THAN DAY 1)	LIQUID MEAL (2 HRS. EARLIER THAN DAY 2)	TULSI TEA	DINNER	LIQUID MEAL	LIQUID MEAL

*A liquid meal can be a shake, a smoothie, or a soup.

As you can see, the illustration clearly indicates whether you will be having a regular solid meal or a liquid meal and when as well as the periods of time when you are not eating. While fasting, you will drink tulsi tea, which you are encouraged to drink between meals as well. Notice also that the timing of your liquid dinner shifts as you move toward the middle of the week, working up to your twenty-four-hour fast starting on day 4. Your liquid dinner should take place earlier each day for the first three days. I will walk you through the day-by-day details in chapter 4.

Determine Your Ayurvedic Dosha

As discussed, I have chosen to include this key Ayurvedic principle as it helps personalize this program to your specific type. It will help you determine which foods to avoid in addition to the Elimination Diet ones, to further intensify and accelerate the detox. Foods also have their own dosha, as it were, or predominant element, which can throw your dosha out of balance. Foods that are fiery will amplify the fire inside, so avoiding them will benefit someone with a predominantly fiery constitution. The effect is cumulative, the more fire you eat, the more your fire will be fed. It is an energetic transaction mostly, not so much a biochemical one, like an allergic reaction mediated by immunoglobulins. This is why the foods-to-avoid list for your dosha is not as strict as the foods-to-avoid list from the Elimination Diet. If you feel too constricted by both, you can be flexible and go ahead with eating a few things from the dosha list of food to avoid, so you don't feel like quitting or not starting at all.

Answer the dosha questionnaire (page 156) twice. The first time base your answers in what is most consistent in your life, the state you have spent most of your life in. The second time base your answers on how you've been feeling more recently, in the past few weeks or months. The first result will indicate your primordial dosha type (your prakriti). The second result will show your current state of imbalance (your vikriti). For CLEAN7 you will use the dosha indicated by your vikriti. If the result shows the same number of answers for two doshas, or the same for the three doshas, you will follow the guidelines for your prakriti. If you are bidoshic or tridoshic you can alternate between the recipes of the two doshas or all of them respectively.

Then turn to your CLEAN7 Dosha-Specific Food Lists (page 158) to understand which foods to avoid.

To make things easy for you once you have determined your current predominant imbalanced dosha, chef James Barry has created three sets of recipes specifically designed for each dosha (pages 194–271).) On the other hand, as long as you follow the guidelines, feel free to make your own dishes. Review the recipes and pick a few that appeal to you, and be sure to have these ingredients on hand before you begin CLEAN7.

In summary: Answer the dosha questionnaire on page 156 twice, once referring to your lifetime (prakriti) and once referring to your present time (vikriti). Follow your vikriti-resulting dosha guideline for CLEAN7. If your vikriti is in balance (no predominant answer for any one single dosha), then do CLEAN7 according to your prakriti.

Get Your Ayurvedic Herbs

Although you can do CLEAN7 without Ayurvedic herbs and get great results, using them will make it work even better. In the graphic of the CLEAN7 protocol on page 59, you'll note that tulsi tea is allowed all day, every day, and you will drink only tulsi tea during your fasting times; however, you can also drink other herbal teas.

Ideally, you will be taking four herbal supplements: tulsi, turmeric, ashwagandha, and triphala. These are Dr. Narendra's favorite detox herbs. Women may want to use shatavari as well, renowned in India for balancing female hormones. If you don't mind additional supplements you can add moringa and brahmi as well. (For a review of all these herbs, go to www.cleanprogram.com/clean7.) I realize this is a lot of supplements, and you may be reluctant to try them all at once or may not be able to afford them. Don't worry, CLEAN7 will give you results without the herbs. Adding the herbs is like pressing your foot on the accelerator. I highly recommend using them. If you must choose one herb only, make it tulsi in capsule form (you will be drinking tulsi tea as well throughout). If you are a woman, and you can add another, make it shatavari. The next one to add is triphala, followed by turmeric, ashwagandha, brahmi, and moringa. That is the ideal order of adding herbs to your program, but they will work regardless of order. You could just use brahmi and moringa and have amazing results.

Tulsi, also known as holy basil, is the only herb that you will be taking both as a supplement and a tea. I suggest you take the herbal supplements with each meal or with tea instead of a meal during fasting times. However, follow the instructions on the label, since the quantity of the herb in each brand's capsule can vary. I recommend the ORGANIC INDIA brand because I know the herbs personally to be genuinely organically grown, as well as planted, harvested, and prepared following authentic Ayurvedic instructions, but there are obviously other brands out there. If you live near a well-stocked health food store or a Whole Foods Market, you should be able to find all the above herbs. If not, all are available on Amazon. For specifics on Ayurvedic herbs, visit www.cleanprogram.com/clean7.

Prepare Your Kitchen—and Your Household

Part of your challenge for the coming week will be to organize your kitchen to make it as easy as possible to prepare your liquid and solid meals. If you are also cooking for your family you may find it easier to have your meal first (or prepare it earlier in the day) so you are not hungry while you prepare a meal for others. Make this challenge part of your commitment to your own goals. After the first couple of days, you will find yourself less hungry and temptation will weaken or even might disappear. Keep in mind that anything you do for yourself ultimately benefits the whole family. Perhaps your partner, roommate, or friend will offer to cook breakfast or dinner a few times during the week—or even offer to detox with you. And don't feel guilty if you occasionally ask others to adapt to accommodate you.

On a more practical note, three countertop appliances come in handy, some or all of which you may already own. A good blender is essential to make the delicious shakes you will be enjoying. A food processor and a multi-cooker (such as an Instapot) facilitate prep and cut cooking time for other recipes. (See page 188 in the introduction to the CLEAN7 recipes.) If you don't already have one or more and are not inclined to invest in them, perhaps you can borrow one from a friend or neighbor. Or simply spend a bit more time prepping veggies and rely on your current pots and pans.

Eliminate Toxic Foods

Review the foods-to-exclude lists for your dosha and the Elimination Diet (page 154) and inventory your refrigerator, freezer, and cabinets. Some foods, such as nightshade family vegetables, are not inherently bad foods; you are simply eliminating them for the time being. But many foods on that list are processed food-like products, full of toxic chemicals. Check the lists of ingredients on the boxes, jars, bags, tubes, and cans of food. They are likely to be full of preservatives, flavor enhancers, stabilizers, colorants, texturizers, and GMOs, and that's just for starters. If you live alone, dispose of them. If your family won't take kindly to an overnight purge of their favorite foods, simply put them on a certain shelf of the fridge, freezer, and pantry and ask for their indulgence for the time being. (For more links to resources on detecting toxic sources in your kitchen, and what to do about it, visit www.cleanprogram/clean7.)

What Are Whole Foods?

For the most part, whole foods are foods as you find them in nature. A whole food can also be organic, but not all whole foods are organic. Plus, the moment vegetables and fruits are processed with added sugar, preservatives, flavor enhancers, and other chemicals, they are no longer whole foods. A pear swimming in a can of sugar syrup no longer qualifies. Nor does a freezer package of stir-fry vegetables in a sauce. On the other hand, "naked" frozen fruit is still a whole food. In general, a whole food is something that contains only what nature produced, but that is not the only criteria upon which to base your dietary choices. For simplicity's sake, let's consider a whole food anything that has not been packaged or processed in any way. Think of it this way, whole foods are what your great-great-grandmother would recognize as food if you could bring her back and take her to a modern supermarket. The CLEAN7 program will give you the best results if you avoid any animal products and do it completely plant based. It also works best for the planet. However, if you won't give them up, the single most important thing to spend money on, even on a tight budget, is organic animal products. When it comes to animal products, it gets more complicated. Toxins accumulate as they go up the food chain. Look for organic, hormone-free pastured chicken and grass-fed meat and choose wild-caught fish over farmed fish. Yes, any chicken breast or a fish filet is a whole food but depending on the life the animal lived before it turned up in the supermarket, it may or may not be something you should consume.

Once you understand which ingredients you'll need for the CLEAN7 solid and liquid meals, figure out where you can buy the healthiest ingredients possible. Check out local farmers' markets, health-food stores, or a supermarket with a good organic selection. Another option is to join a CSA (Community Sponsored Agriculture). Many of them deliver produce grown by local farmers to your door on a weekly basis. Another way to stretch your food dollars is to opt for the organic produce that is most likely to be contaminated with pesticides and buy conventionally grown vegetables and fruits that are least likely to be contaminated. The most important fruits to buy as organic are thin-skinned ones such as peaches, apples, and berries, while you need be less concerned about thick-skinned produce like avocadoes and pineapple, whose skin you remove before eating. The Environmental Working Group is an activist group that has come up with lists of the "The Dirty Dozen" (page 66) and "The Clean Fifteen" (page 67), respectively, which can guide your choices. You can also download wallet-size lists of both at www

.ewg.org. Do the best you can and that your wallet allows. Finally, whether organic or not, be sure to always thoroughly wash your produce with pure water.

Following the CLEAN7 protocol will significantly reduce your body's toxic load. Eating only or primarily whole foods, mostly plants, organic whenever possible—and if you can afford to do so—is the way to go. Once you stop purchasing pricey processed food-like products, you can repurpose some of your hard-earned dollars to spend on organic foods. In addition to the foods you need for CLEAN7, be sure to buy some items that will help you resist cravings, such as raw nuts and herbal teas.

THE CONFUSING WORLD OF ORGANIC FOOD

Most packaged foods are loaded with preservatives that kill bacteria and other microbes as well as additives to give them an appetizing color, scent, and texture. Hydrogenated oils and fats are shelf stable, but these toxic fats can damage your own cells. When you eat a whole foods diet, you omit the preservatives required to extend the shelf life of food-like products that would otherwise spoil. But even most vegetables, fruit, meat, fish, and dairy are "fiddled with" to avoid contamination by bacteria and the resulting product recalls that keep executives in the food, supermarket, and chain restaurant industries up at night. Irradiating food, a technology that extends shelf life, is regarded as an insurance policy against such events, robbing even whole foods of some of their nutritional value and helpful enzymes. Foods that have been irradiated cannot be labeled as USDA Organic.

This label, however, indicates only that no less than 95 percent of the food is organic. Another label, USDA 100 percent Organic, ensures that it is completely organic. Confusing, right?

Continued on next page

Many vegetables and fruits are picked before they are ripe in order to avoid bruising and enable them to travel better without spoiling. When they arrive at their destination, tomatoes, bananas, pears, and a few other fruits are enclosed in a warehouse and blasted with synthetic ethylene gas to hasten the ripening process. If left to ripen on the vine or the tree, these fruits would naturally produce their own ethylene gas. Unlike irradiation, which is an artificial process, because ethylene gas occurs naturally, this warehouse process can be used on food labeled "organic." Whether it was trucked across the country or flown in from another nation, most food—meaning industrial food—is exposed to a toxic stew of fertilizers, pesticides, and insecticides. In our society, looks matter. Some fruits and vegetables may be waxed or treated to other cosmetic procedures to improve their appearance. Piled one upon another, these processes convert much of what you'll find in the average supermarket into poison.

THE DIRTY DOZEN

When conventionally grown, the following foods are most likely to be treated with pesticides, starting with the most heavily contaminated at the top. Try to buy organic versions of these fruits and vegetables.

1. Strawberries
2. Spinach
3. Nectarines
4. Apples
5. Grapes
6. Peaches
7. Cherries
8. Pears
9. Tomatoes
10. Celery
11. Potatoes
12. Sweet bell peppers

THE CLEAN FIFTEEN

When conventionally grown, the following foods are the least likely to be contaminated with pesticides, starting with the least contaminated at the top.

1. Avocados
2. Sweet corn
3. Pineapples
4. Cabbage
5. Onions
6. Sweet peas
7. Papayas
8. Asparagus
9. Mangos
10. Eggplants
11. Honeydew melons
12. Kiwis
13. Cantaloupe melons
14. Cauliflower
15. Broccoli

Start to Journal

Memory is a strange thing. For this reason and so you can see the impact of the CLEAN7 program, I highly recommend you keep a record of your experience, whether on paper or on your computer or electronic notebook, whichever you are most comfortable with and likely to have handy. A recording app on your cell phone is another option.

Before you begin to write in your CLEAN7 journal, take the CLEAN7 audit (page 74). First write down your vision of the new you, your intention, and the results you want to achieve in the following week and beyond. Include any old habits that no longer serve you. You know what they are! List the new habits you plan to replace them with to achieve your full potential. In addition to recording what you have been eating and drinking and how it made you feel, for example, you might also note the times or situations when you have been most subject to temptation by foods that you know are not good for you. Record any of your current symptoms or conditions as a point of reference to see if they change in the future. Some are not likely to improve in a single week, but likely will over time—if you keep clean.

Then over the following week, track your progress, including experiences, emotions, thoughts, or changes in the quality of your sleep. Refer back to your answers to the CLEAN7 audit above and note any changes, as well as any other you observe in your appearance and state of mind. Be sure to log in the detox boosters you engage in each day. Reviewing your journal once you finish the program should help you figure out which diet and lifestyle choices work best for you going forward. Reviewing your journal at a later date might well motivate you to embark on another week on CLEAN7 in the future. (If you decide to stay on CLEAN7 for another week or two, and then gradually reintroduce the foods you eliminated at the start of the program, your journal will help you identify sensitivities to foods you are best avoiding or limiting in the future.)

Take Before Photos

Whether or not you record your progress in a journal, take a selfie or two of yourself before you begin CLEAN7. Shoot it against a plain wall to minimize distractions and keep the focus on you. Paste in your paper journal or add it to your electronic one. Do the same in the middle and at the end of the week, or every day, from the same angle and distance and similar lighting. If you are journaling, paste the photos into your physical or electronic journal. I'll bet that you will be pleasantly surprised at the transformation. Your face and the way your clothes fit will be hard evidence of the difference that CLEAN7 can make in your appearance.

There is no single way to organize and accomplish CLEAN7. If you're not into planning, you may prefer to simply look at the recipes each day and take it day by day. I do advise you to have all the ingredients you will need for the week on hand. Regardless of how you decide to proceed, read this whole chapter, which will prepare you for CLEAN7. If keeping a journal is just not your thing, track only the daily basics using the CLEAN7 planner, discussed below.

Know Your Enemies

You may experience some of the following obstacles when you begin CLEAN7, but once you know which these enemies might be and how to deal with them, you can more easily overcome them.

Hunger

What we call hunger is usually just a feeling we get, more accurately called the "desire to eat." Your body will ask you for the things it is habituated or addicted to, and it will compel you to consume them. This is what people mean when they say, "I'm hungry." Or it may be just the need to comfort, distract, or numb yourself. When this feeling shows up, don't eat; instead, try to take a moment, put your attention on that feeling, and see if you can get to the bottom of it: What is it really? What is the feeling behind it? Usually, when you give it your full attention, the uncomfortable feeling of "hunger" will pass, and you will be more in control of your cravings. Dehydration can also manifest as hunger. Try having a glass of water instead. Take a few breaths, move around a bit, get some fresh air, find something else to occupy your mind.

There are times when you won't want to be bothered with analyzing it. You just need to munch on something. Feel free to snack on whole, fresh foods such as carrot or jicama sticks, celery with hummus, or apple slices topped with almond butter. Nuts, seeds, and olives are all rich in fat and protein, making them satiating and energizing, unlike simple carbs in crackers or rice cakes, which will leave you hungry again after a while. Snacking on any solid food after your liquid dinner will interfere with the fasting window, but tulsi tea is fine. Snacking is allowed but you should know that the less you snack, the stronger your results will be. There is no snacking allowed between dinner and breakfast or during the twenty-four-hour fast period.

Cravings

If you get cravings for sugary, starchy, or dairy foods, you will find that they, along with caffeinated beverages, often lose their appeal once you start CLEAN7. You may have cravings in the first couple of days of the program but pretty soon you will be able to get off that roller coaster of energy highs and lows. Craving toxic food is a classic sign of being in a toxic state. But when you begin to detox, you create a balance that reduces cravings for sugary, starchy, chemical-laden foods. Instead, your body is likely to desire fresh vegetables, fruits, and other real foods. Improving the environment inside the body is much more likely to correct poor eating habits than relying on sheer willpower. When you are fit and healthy, you crave foods that will maintain that state.

That said, disrupting ingrained habits is always challenging, and making changes in what you have eaten and drunk for years is particularly hard. You may find yourself irritable or moody as you begin these changes. Even though the CLEAN7 program addresses these issues both nutritionally and physiologically, you may still find yourself craving the very foods you are trying to eliminate. Again, maximize your chances of success by having good-for-you foods, such as raw nuts and herbal teas, on hand if and when cravings hit.

Social Pressure

Establish a small support system of trusted friends and family members before you begin CLEAN7. As social creatures, we function best with the support of others. Briefly explain what you are doing and why you are comfortable with it. Be clear that you are not asking for permission or approval. You understand and appreciate that they may be concerned but you also expect them to respect your judgment. Don't be surprised if you find that once people find out you are doing a detox program, suddenly you are surrounded by "experts" who offer advice, question what you are doing, or try to convince you that even such a short program with only a single twenty-four-hour fast is a risky endeavor. Most people do not understand what intermittent fasting is and may confuse it with a radical program of drinking only water.

What to do? Don't ask, don't tell, and don't go into a lot of detail. There is no need to share what you are doing with casual friends, acquaintances, or coworkers. What you will be having for lunch most days is a "normal" meal. Plenty of people have smoothies or shakes for breakfast these days so toting one to work for breakfast or an early evening meal shouldn't raise any eyebrows. If you are invited for a pizza or burgers for lunch with coworkers, just say that you have other plans or have brought your meal from home and don't want to waste it but would love to join them another time. Consider starting CLEAN7 on a weekend when you can keep your own schedule and get comfortable with the program before Monday rolls around and you have to integrate it into your work life.

Constipation

Your bowels will do some heavy lifting this week, hopefully. If not, something is wrong. Good bowel movements are always crucial, but especially during a detox program. Do everything in your power to support daily bowel movements.

Blending roughage in the form of kale, chard, and other leafy greens into your liquid meals helps ensure that you have regular bowel movements.

Another approach to constipation is to simply get more active. Hopping up and down on a trampoline or jumping rope actually helps keep "things moving." So does taking long walks and practicing yoga, thanks to the twisting and toning of your body both inside and out. Lying on your back and hugging your knees to your chest is an especially helpful posture, as is simply squatting. Your yoga teacher can suggest other poses or check them out online. If you do need to use a laxative, make sure it is a natural one. My favorite is Dr. Schulze's Intestinal Formula #1. Magnesium in supplement form also helps; magnesium powder is the most effective. Take a hot bath, read a book, or maybe watch something funny on television, as laughter helps reduce stress and releases colon muscles. Try to wake up an hour or two before you need to be anywhere in the morning and drink two glasses of hot or warm water with lemon. Having daily bowel movements is really important. If you go a day without any, consider having a colonic that day or the next. I have found that self-administering devices, such as the Implant-O-Rama, are very useful to have on hand (www.implantorama.com). For more solutions for constipation visit www.cleanprogram.com/clean7.

Headaches

During the coming week, you may experience withdrawal symptoms as a result of eliminating certain foods and beverages, particularly sugar, caffeine, and alcohol, as well as a host of chemicals in processed foods. Headaches may occur mostly during the first day or two of the program. Instead of taking any over-the-counter medications such as Advil, ride out the headaches. They will pass.

However, if you can't tough it out, lie down or take a nap. Magnesium helps with headaches as well as constipation. Or take a walk or do yoga or some stretching exercises. Massage or acupuncture can work wonders for a headache. While taking an over-the-counter drug may provide short-term relief, the headache may return with a vengeance once the drug wears off, plus medications only add more toxins to your body.

Bad Dreams, Irritability, and Mood Changes

When you encourage the body to release toxins, as you are doing with CLEAN7, you also detox quantum toxins of stress and anxiety, including stuck negative emotions from past trauma. It is not uncommon to experience either bad dreams or nasty emotions, don't worry; they will pass. Just make sure you don't off-load on innocent bystanders.

Also, be prepared for occasional moments when your resolve to complete CLEAN7 may waver. That is perfectly normal. Don't judge yourself for having such thoughts. Just remember to tap into your original desire and keep on going. CLEAN7 is a process and a single moment of weakness such as having a glass of wine or a baked potato is not a reason to call it quits. Yes, it is a step backward, but all you need to do is get back on track and keep going. The very fact that you regard this as a lapse is proof that you want to change, which is a positive thing. Hold on to that thought and recommit to staying true to the program for the rest of the week.

Boredom, Impatience, and Noncompliance

- *Boredom/Impatience:* If you feel much better, less toxic, and less bloated before completing CLEAN7, you may be wondering, "Do I really need to hang in another 48 hours?" Yes, hang in. I designed CLEAN7 to achieve great results in seven days.

You may be feeling significantly better, but you won't know how much better you can feel unless you just hang in there for a couple of days longer.

- *Noncompliance:* What if despite your best intentions, life intervenes. Perhaps an emotional upset throws you for a loop, and you fall off the CLEAN7 wagon. Let's say that happens on day 5. All you have to do is just repeat day 5 and take it from there. Don't waste a minute blaming yourself. Alternatively, if you decide to make up your own CLEAN7 by eating solid meals when liquid meals are specified or eating foods on the foods-to-avoid list, you may be getting some results, but not the results that I can reliably predict if you follow the program to the letter. So, here's some tough love: If you veer away from these principles, you may want to take a break and repeat the program properly in a few weeks with a different mindset.

THE CLEAN7 AUDIT

The following questions will help you get a handle on your level of toxicity, as indicated by your "yes" answers.

- Do you have headaches?
- Do you frequently catch colds or viruses?
- Are you constipated?
- Do you often have diarrhea?
- Are your eyes and nose itchy or watery at certain times of year?
- Do you have allergies or hay fever?
- Are you often congested or "mucusy"?
- Do you feel bloated after eating?
- Are you unable to shed extra weight despite eating less and exercising?

- Is your face or are parts of your body puffy?
- Do you have dark circles under your eyes?
- Do you regularly get heartburn?
- Are you often flatulent?
- Do you burp a lot?
- Do you have bad breath or B.O.?
- Do you have a thin white coating on the back of your tongue in the morning?
- Do you crave sugary, starchy, or dairy foods?
- Are you a restless sleeper?
- Do you have itchy skin, pimples, or another skin condition?
- Are your joints or muscles painful or stiff?
- Do you take several prescription medications?
- Do you often feel low, apathetic, or tired?
- Are you forgetful or do you have difficulty concentrating?
- Do you often get angry or frustrated?

All these conditions may well be symptoms of toxicity and indications that doing the CLEAN7 program is exactly what you need to begin the process of removing physical (and emotional) toxins from your body (and mind). Other clear signals include an especially high sensitivity to odors such as perfumes, cleaning fluids, gasoline, personal care products, and additives in processed foods. If you are exposed to potentially toxic chemicals in your home or workplace, you almost certainly need to do detox programs more frequently. I also strongly advise you to eliminate or minimize such exposure (for links to info on detoxing your home visit www.cleanprogram.com/clean7).

The previous questions may have been a real eye opener. For example, did you know that toxic buildup can affect your emo-

Continued on next page

tions or your ability to concentrate? Or that some prescription and OTC medications include toxic ingredients that accumulate in your body? Or that headaches and restless sleep could be tied to toxicity?. If you really need OTC medications, check if what you need is available from companies like Genexa (www .genexa.com) that make cleaner versions of the most commonly used ones.

A PRE-CLEANSE, OR NOT?

If you had mostly "no" responses to the CLEAN audit, chances are you are already eating and living relatively clean. However, if you answered "yes" to four or more of the questions above, I highly recommend doing a short pre-cleanse to first avoid more intense withdrawals. To do so, omit all or most of the following foods and beverages for the next three days, and then begin CLEAN7 on the following day. This will make everything go smoother during the program and even allow it to go deeper.

- Caffeine (unless it comes in matcha, yerba maté, or green tea)
- Alcohol
- Sugar
- All dairy products
- Eggs
- Processed oils such as canola
- White rice, wheat, corn, barley, spelt, kamut, rye, triticale, and oats
- Grapefruit, oranges, and orange juice

- Nightshade vegetables: tomatoes, eggplant, peppers, potatoes
- Ideally all meats but at minimum all processed meats
- Shrimp and other shellfish
- Soybeans and soy products
- Peanuts

CLEAN7 Tip: Consider doing the program with a spouse, partner, or good friend. You'll be able to support and encourage each other, increasing the chances of success for both of you. A larger group is even better, since intentions that are aligned potentiate one another. I've seen many yoga classes team up and do it together as well as entire departments in certain companies. This is a great, fun way to do it.

CLEAN7 Tip: Line Up Your Network

If you are planning to have at least one colonic or a massage while detoxing, do some homework so you can make appointments *before* you begin CLEAN7. If either of these detox boosters are new to you, get recommendations from friends or health professionals or look online to find pros in your area. The same applies to finding a place to have a sauna. Don't leave this until the last minute or you are unlikely to be able to enjoy these benefits in a timely fashion. Cryotherapy, exposing oneself to freezing temperatures for a few minutes, is something that can boost your program as well. Places that offer cryotherapy are becoming more popular. Chances are there is one somewhere close to you.

Get Ready for Great Results

Here are some of the benefits you can expect:

Mental Clarity

Something amazing happens when you start eliminating ama, your accumulated toxicity, from your body. Its lower vibrational frequency attracts lower vibrational thoughts and emotions. As the load begins to get reduced, there will be more space for clear thoughts, as well as creative ones. As inflammation and other adaptive processes wind down, the energy that is freed from them also contributes to enhanced mental agility. In addition, the intermittent fasting state will further sharpen your senses and give you the lightness that you would need if you were living in the wild and had to hunt for your next meal. Your ambition gets stronger, which can be redirected into anything that you want to accomplish.

Equanimity

Defined as "calmness of mind, composure, evenness of temper," this promise of equanimity is a biggie. And this is exactly what can happen. I think of the CLEAN7 program as biochemical and physiologic yoga. Just like yoga, the CLEAN7 program is based on ancient Eastern wisdom. And just as yoga balances the mind through physical shifts that activate beneficial nervous pathways leading to a calmer mind, the CLEAN7 program does it through physiologic shifts that lead to an inner cellular-biochemical environment that promotes the same. The brain in your gut will redirect its focus from adaptation and survival activities into ones that result in better production of serotonin and balancing of other neurotransmitters.

Emotions are a large component of cleansing so you may feel

more emotional, perhaps crying more easily than usual while doing CLEAN7. For most of us, food doesn't just satisfy physical hunger, it also feeds our emotional needs. That's why you reach for the
cookie jar when you are exhausted or bored or crave ice cream after
a breakup. Once you understand these motivations, you will be better equipped to eliminating the hold that toxic emotions have over
you and your choices.

Weight Loss

I once met a spiritual teacher who was famous for giving his fol-
lowers expensive gifts. When asked why he did that he answered,
"I give people what they want in the hope that they will eventually
want what I really have to give them." I feel the same way about
the CLEAN7 program. The reality is that many of us want to lose
weight, regardless if it is for health reasons or not. So yes, CLEAN7
is a great way to lose weight. And there are many reasons for that.
Part of the accumulation of ama is mucus that is formed to buffer
toxic molecules. This mucus is a sponge that retains water and gets
stuck within and between cells. This is the cause of the puffiness in
your skin. This mucus will start to shed away and with it the water
it retained. You may find yourself urinating way more often than
regularly, more even than you would expect when drinking more
water. This causes a significant amount of weight loss and reduction
of the puffiness. This is how you may lose a whole dress size or two
in seven days or fit in jeans that were too tight for years. And this
is why your skin glows and you look better and younger. Another
big reason is that the immune system in your gut starts to relax and
shrink in size, just as a muscle that is all pumped up from lifting
heavy weights shrinks when it's well rested. Since 80 percent of our
immune system is within and around your intestines, it can get
pretty bulgy when hyperactive. When you see a person with skinny
or normal legs and arms but a protruding belly, this is what is go-

ing on. The immune system is lifting weights. And you are about to give it a week's vacation. The bulge in your belly will get significantly less tight and smaller. This translates to a lot of weight. It is okay to do the CLEAN7 program just to lose weight. It is okay if you do it to fit into your wedding dress and look great for the wedding pictures. I'll bet you big time that you won't want to let go of how it feels, along with the overall effects in your life. My friend Farzad was doing just fine. He had no symptoms or any problems that he was aware of. But when I saw him in his bathing suit, I pointed out his inflated belly. I told him he needs to do my program. He said, "No way, I don't have twenty-one days for that." I told him about CLEAN7 and he jumped right in. A week later he called me to thank me and tell me that not only had he lost eleven pounds, but he had a jolt of energy, he was fitting into pants that he hadn't for a long time, and that it had already paid off in his work. What he liked the most was his experience of being in the fasting state. He decided to make it a part of his life going forward.

Energy Surges

You may experience a jolt of energy or even feel a bit jittery by the middle of the week doing CLEAN7. You might not fall asleep as easily as you're accustomed to doing or may wake up earlier than usual. Resist the urge to take a sleeping pill. Limiting your food intake and minimizing digestion time with more liquid meals has liberated energy, but your body may not quite know what to do with it yet. In the meantime, put it to good work by going for a walk or a run. Or get to some of those chores you've been putting off. Read a book or write those long-overdue emails. Take advantage of this temporary shift in energy allocation. Soon things will fall into place and equilibrium will return. On the other hand, if sleep deprivation is interfering with your life, try magnesium supplementation to help relax.

Deeper Sleep

Digesting and assimilating food can interfere with getting a good night's sleep. But by day 3 or 4 on CLEAN7, you are likely to find you that you are sleeping more deeply. In addition to the shorter digestion and assimilation time needed to process liquid meals for dinner, each day you will have your dinner shake earlier than the day before. This means that by the time you climb into bed, you may well be already almost done with digestion, which promises a deeper restorative sleep. You are also more likely to dream in this state and to recall your dreams.

Beauty

So many aches and pains go away during CLEAN7 and so many more serious symptoms start improving that it is impossible to list them all, but the thing that I get so much gratitude about when I put people on CLEAN7 is how much better they look. Their skin glows, their hair shines, their nails become stronger. Beware, CLEAN7 can make you even sexier than you already are!

The Right Time

When is the right time to embark on what could be a life-changing experience? The first time, choose a week without business travel, family reunions, or any other celebratory stressful personal or work-related situations. The week your mother-in-law is visiting is probably not the best time! On the other hand, don't keep delaying, waiting for the perfect time. It doesn't exist. After the first time, every time you do the CLEAN7 program you will get better at incorporating it to your regular life, to the point that it becomes seamless.

No matter how busy you are, you would make time for your

child's birthday party or complete that rush project that your boss just dropped on your desk, right? Make time for CLEAN7 in the same way. It is a good idea to start on a weekend when you have more control over your personal life. It also gives you a couple of days to get familiar with the program during the initial days that require the most adjustment from your normal routine. (If your job involves working on weekends, adjust accordingly.) Trying to do CLEAN7 while you are changing jobs, moving, or going through an emotional crisis such as a breakup is probably not the best time, although there are people who almost always need such a kick in the pants to finally get motivated.

Once you find the best time, block it out on your calendar just as you would any social or business commitment. Now that you have committed to a certain time frame, it is essential that you have everything you need on hand before you start. Finding your fridge is empty on day 4 is not going to serve your interests.

In addition to assembling the food and supplements you will need, scan the planner on page 145 or download it at www.clean program.com/clean7, and list the meals you are planning to make, along with any ingredients you need to purchase as well as the supplements and herbs you will be using. Post the planner on your refrigerator door or another place in plain sight. Unlike your journal, which is for your eyes only, the planner is out in the open as a constant reminder of what you plan to do each day.

In the following chapter, I'll provide a detailed day-by-day description of everything you need to successfully complete the CLEAN7 program.

4

The CLEAN7 Program Day by Day

Welcome to the CLEAN7 program. I congratulate you on making the decision to embark on this journey. Now that you understand why detoxification is so important to your physical and emotional well-being, as well as what to expect in the coming days, and you've gathered what you need, it's finally time to get into the day-by-day details of the program. The graphic on page 85 is just a peek at what's to come. In this chapter, you'll learn *what* and *when* to eat. I'll hold your hand every step of the way, alerting you of what to expect throughout the week and introducing you to multiple ways to enhance your detox. CLEAN7 has a particular arc that you will experience over the seven-day period as you work up to a twenty-four-hour fast, during which you drink only herbal tea and water and then gently return to the meal pattern on day 1 as your last day: shake-lunch-shake.

Here is a brief overview:

- Most days you will have a shake for both breakfast and dinner. A shake is liquid food that doesn't need as much digestive work as solid food does and is absorbed more quickly. The whole process of digestion and absorption is eased and shortened—think of shakes as fuel injection—so you will enter the detoxification process sooner and stay in it for longer. In that way you maximize the intensity of detoxification, compared to what follows a solid meal.

- You will eat solid food only at lunchtime following your CLEAN7 dosha diet. Some days a smaller meal, or snack, will be your lunch.

- You will build up to a twenty-four-hour fast by extending the window between dinner one day and breakfast the following day over four days from about twelve hours to about eighteen hours. Next you will fast for twenty-four hours and then return to a twelve-hour window over the last two days. I will walk you through the specifics of each day, each time, starting with the graphic opposite, highlighting the day in question. The CLEAN7 program itself is extremely effective, but there are a number of "boosters" that make detox even deeper and more fun. Rest and sleep (see page 102), movement (see page 94), saunas and hot and cold plunges (see page 88), colonics and enemas (see page 91), massage and acupuncture (see page 99), meditation (see page 96), and simply having fun will all boost the results of CLEAN7. You'll find information on these detox boosters within the instructions for each day. I strongly suggest you review the booster content *before* you begin the program. Ideally you would engage in *each one* of these, once a day in many cases, or one or more times in the week in other cases. So, take a close look at all of them to consider which ones you plan to do and when and where you plan to do them. The more of these booster practices you engage in, the better your detox will be. As a bonus, the boosters also increase the likelihood that you will lose some inches and pounds in the week to come.

Day 1 of CLEAN7

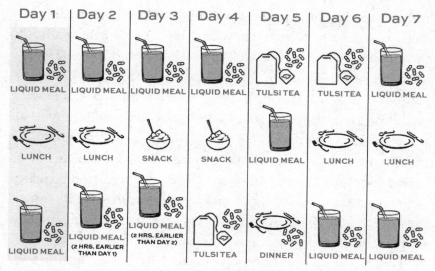

A liquid meal can be a shake, a smoothie, or a soup.

Day 1 is the hardest day of CLEAN7 for many. Today you suddenly disrupt deeply ingrained habits. Not easy. But I have seen people in all walks of life and in all kinds of circumstances complete the program successfully. And so can you. I will provide the guidance, but you must deliver on the resolve. You're going to begin the first day of CLEAN7 with a shake for breakfast, then a solid meal for lunch, and another shake for dinner. If you believe the premise that breakfast is the most important meal of the day and you usually eat a big one, this change may be a bit difficult initially. Same thing if you are accustomed to eating a large dinner. According to Ayurvedic Medicine, the biggest meal of the day should be lunch, when the *agni*, the fire of digestion, is at its greatest strength. When you eat a big breakfast, you're putting your digestive system to work, actually slowing you down rather than giving you the strength to do what you need to do each day, whether it's caring for your kids or dealing with your daily work-load. Once you become accustomed to a liquid breakfast, you'll realize that drinking it makes you feel lighter and more mentally clear, energetic, and productive. In fact, a lot of people who do the CLEAN7 program wind up having a shake for breakfast long term. Choose from one of Chef James Barry's delicious shakes, or-ganized by dosha (pages 194–255), or create your own, following your dosha guidelines (pages 158–163). The shakes will provide all the nutrients needed to carry you through to lunch and will do so without making your digestive system work hard. You will be taking some or all of the following Ayurvedic herbal supplements with your breakfast: tulsi, triphala, turmeric, ashwagandha, mor-inga, brahmi, plus shatavari if you are a woman. (Again, you will find information on them at www.cleanprogram.com/clean7.)

Lunch will be your only solid meal of the day, following your dosha diet as well. It's a good idea to post your dosha's list of foods to avoid on your refrigerator door. Check out the recipes for deli-cious meal options on pages 194–271, which are arranged by dosha. Or use your own recipes, following the guidelines for your dosha. A few more essentials:

- Stay hydrated throughout the day with filtered water and tulsi tea or other herbal teas.

- In addition to having the tea and the liquid in your shakes, make sure you drink plenty of water to help flush out toxins. If you are not urinating once an hour, you are not drinking enough water. You should drink only filtered, pure water, not tap water, which likely contains toxic chemicals. (See page 181.)

Your dinner will consist of another shake. Today you can have your shake whenever you usually eat dinner. Have your evening Ayurvedic herbal supplements with this meal. Have the same shake you had for breakfast, swap out some different veggies or fruits, or sample a new recipe. Feel free to have tulsi tea or another herbal tea after your dinner shake but no solid food.

CLEAN7 provides the amount of food you need to feel full and fueled with plenty of energy, even though much of it is in liquid form. Most of us consume a lot of food, but don't get adequate nutrients. Depending on what you were eating before you started this program, you may be more or less nutrient starved. During CLEAN7 both the quantity of food and nutrients in your shakes and in your one solid meal are more than adequate to keep you nourished.

CLEAN7 Tip: If you have a pair of jeans or another item of clothing that is a little too snug for comfort, try it on today and take a picture to add to your journal. Then try on those same jeans on day 7 and compare.

CLEAN7 Tip: If your mornings are hectic, make your shake the night before, refrigerate it, and drink it before you leave the house. Another time saver: double the recipe for your morning shake and reserve half for your liquid evening meal.

Booster #1: Sweating

Nature would not have included the function of sweating if it was not necessary. Judging by the fact that the skin is the body's largest organ and the vehicle through which we perspire, sweating must be important. We have come to understand that sweating helps reduce the body's temperature through evaporation, a way of eliminating certain toxins, and this function is intimately connected to the nervous and emotional systems. That's why we start sweating when we get nervous. If the "sweating apparatus" is never used, it atrophies, just as a muscle that is still for a long time does. It is important to sweat periodically. If you are in the habit of breaking a sweat through exercise, you are good. If not, I highly recommend you put this muscle to work some other way. A great way of doing so is with saunas.

Saunas

Saunas have been around for a long time. The Finns were on to the health benefits of saunas two thousand years ago! Infrared saunas are the most efficient for detox. This relatively new technology heats your body rather than heating the air through convection as a traditional Finnish sauna does. An infrared sauna creates radiant heat from light waves in the infrared spectrum. They penetrate more deeply below the skin than the heat of a regular sauna, exciting the fat molecules to vibrate and enabling them to release toxins. Spending time in a sauna also boosts circulation, which is desirable at all times, but especially during CLEAN7, helping the blood carry toxins efficiently to the liver for processing. Among the other benefits of sauna time are relaxation, improved sleep, and relief from sore muscles. Still another benefit is glowing skin. If you are used to traditional saunas, you will probably find that the infrared type makes you sweat more despite the lower temperature, even more if it's a far infrared sauna. In either case, be sure to drink plenty of pure water during and after the sauna. It is safe to take a sauna every day until you break a good sweat, particularly while you are doing CLEAN7. My favorite far infrared saunas are the Sunlighten saunas (www.sunlighten.com). I have one at home and use it every day. A quick Google search will find the nearest one that you can pay to use. Steam rooms can be helpful as well.

Alternating Hot and Cold

Hot and cold plunges are a detox secret weapon. Repeatedly alternating between extremes of water temperature boosts circulation and detoxification. As your largest organ, your skin contains miles of blood-filled arterioles and venules, which relax and dilate with heat and contract with cold. When this alternating relax-contract pattern is stimulated, your skin pumps almost as much blood as your heart does. You don't need to go to a spa or bathhouse to do it. Instead, just turn on the water in your shower as hot as you can tolerate it for one minute and then as cold as you can tolerate for another minute. Repeat four or five times.

As I wrote this book, I took time out every day to break a sweat in an infrared sauna and then jump in a cold pool, repeating it three or four times. I felt great.

Day 2 of CLEAN7

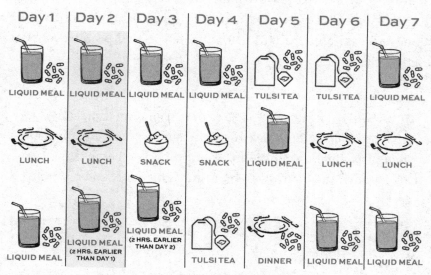

Day 1	Day 2	Day 3	Day 4	Day 5	Day 6	Day 7
LIQUID MEAL	LIQUID MEAL	LIQUID MEAL	LIQUID MEAL	TULSI TEA	TULSI TEA	LIQUID MEAL
LUNCH	LUNCH	SNACK	SNACK	LIQUID MEAL	LUNCH	LUNCH
LIQUID MEAL	LIQUID MEAL (2 HRS. EARLIER THAN DAY 1)	LIQUID MEAL (2 HRS. EARLIER THAN DAY 2)	TULSI TEA	DINNER	LIQUID MEAL	LIQUID MEAL

*A liquid meal can be a shake, a smoothie, or a soup.

Day 2 will be very similar to day 1 with one small but significant difference; you will have your evening liquid dinner earlier than on day 1. Make yourself another delicious dosha-appropriate shake for breakfast, following a recipe on pages 194–255, or your own creation. Take your morning Ayurvedic herbal supplements with your breakfast shake. When lunchtime rolls around, choose a dosha-suitable recipe or make your own meal, again following your dosha diet.

Today you are going to increase the window between your last shake of the day and the first shake tomorrow morning, ideally by two hours, for a total of fourteen hours between the two meals. This means that if you had your evening shake at 8:00 p.m. on the first day, have it today at 6:00 p.m. Take your Ayurvedic herbal supplements with your evening shake. If you are keeping a journal, note the time at which you had dinner, as well as any detox boosters you engaged in today. When you tuck yourself into bed, remind yourself that you've done your body a big favor by ensuring that much of the work of digestion and assimilation will be done earlier than the night before, which should promise a better night's sleep.

CLEAN7 Tip: If you are unable to have your dinner shake as early as advised, delay breakfast the next morning for a comparable amount of time. Avoid the habit of eating late because the later your dinner, the more digestion intrudes on detox and restorative sleep.

The Question of Snacking

Snacking is permitted on the CLEAN7 program, but if you do get the urge, try drinking a glass of pure water before you have a snack. Dehydration can mimic the sensation of hunger. Do some deep breathing, go outside, or move around the house. What you thought was hunger will likely soon pass and you will have triumphed over your cravings. The Ayurvedic herbs and herbal supplements you are taking will help regulate peaks and lows of insulin, thereby eliminating cravings as well as enhancing fat burning.

Typically, by the time you complete CLEAN7, sugar cravings tend to go down. CLEAN7 will shed light on your habits, eating patterns, and emotional and physical triggers. Eliminating toxins also encourages the growth of healthy microflora in your digestive tract. Consuming more greens in both your solid meals and particularly in your liquid ones, by blending them in, often encourages a healthy balance that helps reduce sugar cravings.

Booster #2: Colonics

Colonic hydrotherapy, aka a colonic, boosts the removal of waste from your intestines. Many Western-trained physicians are skeptical of the benefits of colonics or worry that they are not safe. Not true. Many decades ago there were colon hydrotherapy rooms in many hospitals in America. They are beneficial when administered by an experienced therapist. During a colonic, pure water under low pressure is introduced into the colon and then withdrawn. This irrigation assists in releasing waste. Both open and closed systems are hygienic, discreet, and not uncomfortable; you can research which you prefer. Colonics are most beneficial while on a detox program. Enemas are a self-administered way of irrigating the lower colon and are also helpful when detoxing. Enema self-administration devices such as the Implant-O-Rama (implant orama.com), which works as well as a colonic with a more sophisticated device and way better than a simple enema by gravity bag, can be incredibly useful.

Day 3 of CLEAN7

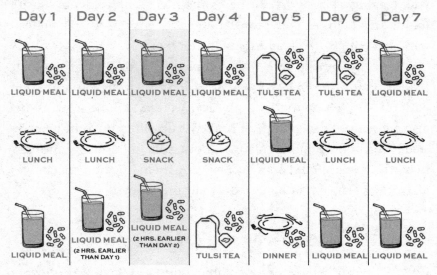

Day 1	Day 2	Day 3	Day 4	Day 5	Day 6	Day 7
LIQUID MEAL	LIQUID MEAL	LIQUID MEAL	LIQUID MEAL	TULSI TEA	TULSI TEA	LIQUID MEAL
LUNCH	LUNCH	SNACK	SNACK	LIQUID MEAL	LUNCH	LUNCH
LIQUID MEAL	LIQUID MEAL (2 HRS. EARLIER THAN DAY 1)	LIQUID MEAL (2 HRS. EARLIER THAN DAY 2)	TULSI TEA	DINNER	LIQUID MEAL	LIQUID MEAL

*A liquid meal can be a shake, a smoothie, or a soup.

By day 3 you should be getting used to your new diet, to eating less often and allowing more time between meals. You should be proud of the strength of your resolve. By three days into CLEAN7 your body is adapting as it reclaims energy from digestion and begins some serious detox work. If your systems were out of whack earlier, this shift can feel odd. Your sleep patterns, frequency and nature of your bowel movements, your appetite, and even your emotions are experiencing changes. Be open to these changes and just go with them. They are only temporary. Change is happening and your body is adapting. Accommodate it.

Thanks to the nutritious shakes you have been having for breakfast and dinner, you probably aren't missing whatever you were accustomed to having for breakfast before you began CLEAN7. If you were not able to have your dinner shake last night two hours earlier, have this morning's shake later. If necessary, you can take your shake with you if you work outside the home to ensure that fourteen hours have elapsed since your shake the evening before.

To avoid boredom, consider trying a new dosha-suitable shake today from the recipes on pages 194–255 or experiment with a new one of your own. As usual, take your Ayurvedic herbal supplements with the shake. You'll be making two additional changes to your CLEAN7 program today. First of all, instead of lunch, you will be having a snack. Call it a mini-lunch if that makes it more palatable. Basically, it's half the amount of yesterday's lunch. (You'll note that our meal recipes provide servings sizes for a snack as well as a meal. Specifically, a snack portion is half that of a meal.)

Today's second change: from the time you finished your dinner shake on day 2 until your shake this morning, you went for fourteen hours without eating. Now you are going to ramp it up to sixteen hours. Do this by moving your dinner shake up two hours earlier, even if this means having it in the late afternoon. Add some yummy additions to make your shake extra filling and nutritious and don't forget to take your Ayurvedic herbal supplements with it. Resist any impulse to have a snack after your dinner shake. As always, you can have tulsi tea and/or other herbal teas, during the day and after your evening/late afternoon shake.

If you are keeping a journal, jot down how you are feeling, any problems you are encountering, any breakthroughs you have made over the last three days, and the detox boosters you engaged in today.

CLEAN7 Tip: If you may be having your second shake of the day while you are not at home, make a double batch in the morning and take the second serving with you in a thermos.

Booster #3: Detox with Exercise, Movement, and More

Exercise or just simple movement boosts elimination. It increases blood and lymph circulation, makes you sweat, and even stimulates your bowels. Exercise also makes bowel movements easier to pass by decreasing the time it takes food to move through the large intestine. Activity also makes you breathe more deeply and accelerates your heart rate, which stimulates the natural contraction of intestinal muscles, again assisting with bowel movements. It's a great way to break a sweat and activate that important function that most of us never even use.

Exercise also relaxes your mind and pulls you into the present, as anyone who has experienced what athletes commonly call "the zone" knows. Activity burns calories, and releases endorphins, the feel-good hormones that are nature's antidotes to stress. If you are already active, you can continue to be so during CLEAN7. However, cleansing is intense work, so show your body some extra love by resting more than usual. Second, don't run a marathon while cleansing, and avoid any intense fitness training, especially in the first few days. Remember, the more you work out, the more you need to recover. In exercise and recovery mode, energy moves to those affected areas and away from the detoxification processes, much as the process of digestion interferes with detoxification. Pushing yourself to maintain an intense workout routine actually hinders the detox program by adding to your body's workload. Consider cutting your workouts in half if you have an intense routine. On the other hand, you may find that you can maintain your energy level while detoxing. Some people find it actually increases. If so, fine, but overall, listen to your body and pay close attention to any changes, adjusting as necessary.

If you have a very active routine and feel fine maintaining it, boost your food intake slightly. Rather than snacking, slightly increase your intake of both liquid and solid meals. Add a bit more fat and protein to your meals and shakes and your body will burn that fuel more efficiently, and you'll remain both satiated and energized.

On the other hand, if you are feeling more tired than usual, stay with light activities such as walking, gentle yoga, or some sit-ups, push-ups, and other body-weight exercises. All enable you to stay active, tone your muscles (which leads to increased fat burning and efficient energy use), and stimulate the detox process. Do something every day, even if it's just making the commitment to walk more and take the stairs whenever you can. At the minimum, try to move for twenty minutes a day. And remember, playing with your kids counts! Exercise needn't be work. Take a cue from how they engage in the simple pleasures of climbing, jumping, twisting, rolling around, and tossing a ball. Play is a great stress reliever and will only add to the program.

Don't stop there. I encourage you to activate the right brain by expressing your creative side, perhaps by dancing, singing, playing an instrument, painting, sculpting, gardening, writing poetry, or whatever inspires you.

Day 4 of CLEAN7

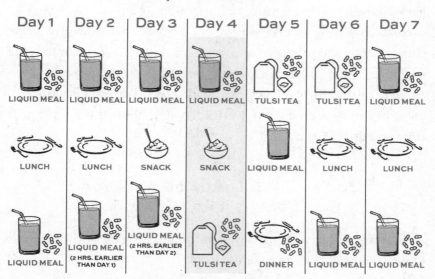

Day 1	Day 2	Day 3	Day 4	Day 5	Day 6	Day 7
LIQUID MEAL	LIQUID MEAL	LIQUID MEAL	LIQUID MEAL	TULSI TEA	TULSI TEA	LIQUID MEAL
LUNCH	LUNCH	SNACK	SNACK	LIQUID MEAL	LUNCH	LUNCH
LIQUID MEAL	LIQUID MEAL (2 HRS. EARLIER THAN DAY 1)	LIQUID MEAL (2 HRS. EARLIER THAN DAY 2)	TULSI TEA	DINNER	LIQUID MEAL	LIQUID MEAL

A liquid meal can be a shake, a smoothie, or a soup.

Once you wake up well rested on day 4, get ready. This is the day your twenty-four-hour fast starts. Today you will be fasting from the time you finish your lunchtime snack/mini meal until lunch with a shake tomorrow. Make your morning shake really succulent by adding some extra green, leafy vegetables. Boost the fat content with some avocado, almonds if your dosha allows, or a dosha-appropriate oil. Take your Ayurvedic herbal supplements with your shake as usual.

At lunchtime, you'll have a snack/small lunch. You will not be eating any food after this meal until your shake for lunch on day 5, meaning for at least twenty-four hours, during which time you will truly enter the fasting state. You will have tulsi tea and/ or another herbal tea for dinner along with your Ayurvedic herbal supplements, as well as more tea later in the evening, if you wish.

Arguably, this is the most difficult day of the seven-day program. One way to help yourself get through what may seem like a long day is to find something to distract you at the time when you would normally be eating and on into the evening. That could mean settling down with a good book, playing Scrabble, doing a jigsaw puzzle, seeing a film, or just catching up on your favorite sitcom—anything to take your mind off food. Alternatively, make this the day when you have a massage, spend half an hour in a sauna, or attend a yoga class, all powerful detox boosters. Even though distracting yourself can work great, sitting with the discomfort can be even more powerful. Try it, if not this time, the next time you do CLEAN7.

Booster #4: Detox Mentally and Emotionally with Meditation

A daily meditation of just seven minutes can give you incredible benefits. Check chapter 5 for details.

Day 5 of CLEAN7

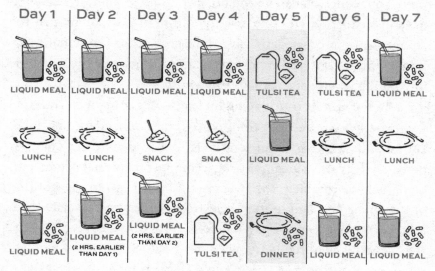

Day 1	Day 2	Day 3	Day 4	Day 5	Day 6	Day 7
LIQUID MEAL	LIQUID MEAL	LIQUID MEAL	LIQUID MEAL	TULSI TEA	TULSI TEA	LIQUID MEAL
LUNCH	LUNCH	SNACK	SNACK	LIQUID MEAL	LUNCH	LUNCH
LIQUID MEAL	LIQUID MEAL (2 HRS. EARLIER THAN DAY 1)	LIQUID MEAL (2 HRS. EARLIER THAN DAY 2)	TULSI TEA	DINNER	LIQUID MEAL	LIQUID MEAL

A liquid meal can be a shake, a smoothie, or a soup.

When you wake up on day 5, you are going to feel great, but you'll probably really want a breakfast shake as well. Hang in there a little longer as you focus mind over matter. You are doing great. Instead of your usual morning shake, have a cup of tulsi tea along with your Ayurvedic herbal supplements. As you sip your tea, comfort yourself with the realization that you are almost done with your twenty-four-hour fast. In just a few hours, you will be enjoying your first meal of the day. At lunch you will have a shake, to break the fast gently. This is the only day in which you will have a shake for lunch, and it may be inconvenient if you are working. But this one is important. Prepare your shake beforehand and take it with you if you can't prepare it at work.

Congratulations! You have overcome the two most difficult days on CLEAN7. Or perhaps it wasn't all that difficult after all. I'll bet you feel proud—and also *clean*. Drink slowly and savor every sip of your lunch shake. As you do, give some thought to what you have just experienced. Your twenty-four-hour fast potentiated the detoxification processes and gave you a taste of the hormonal, emotional, and overall health benefits of a fast. It may be the first time in your life when your gut felt truly empty.

When you start introducing intermittent fasting into your life, you experience a freedom from our cultural dependence on food. Eating and thinking about food need not rule your life—or your body. There is also a great sense of accomplishment that comes with being able to complete the twenty-four-hour fast—to say nothing of the whole program. I often hear from people that it made them aware of not needing to eat that much to function really well, or that they actually feel even better when they eat less. Now is when you might even be thinking, "Hey, I could do this for another week!"

Now that you are nearing the end of the program, you will start transitioning back to the shake-lunch-shake schedule. This evening for the first time this week, you can have a solid food dinner. Choose a recipe appropriate for your dosha on pages 194–271 or make a favorite recipe of your own. Take your Ayurvedic herbal supplements. If you're doing CLEAN7 with a partner, this would be a great opportunity to get together for a delicious and CLEAN7-compliant meal to cheer each other on and compare notes about what's been happening over the previous five days.

Now that you have experienced fasting, I hope you are feeling the benefits. Your body should be feeling comfortable and energetic. Your mind is likely to be clearer as well. You may be wondering why we don't let ourselves feel this way more often. Now that you know how to create this clean, clear state of mind and body, you can do it again whenever you want to.

Booster #5: Detox with Massage and Acupuncture

That post-massage feeling of relaxation, renewal, and release from stress is complete bliss. Like fasting, massage is an ancient practice used by societies worldwide to address both mental and physical ailments. By manipulating your muscles, fascia, connective tissue, tendons, and ligaments, massage helps regulate hormones, enhance immunity, lower blood pressure, and reduce muscle pain. Importantly, massage also helps to detoxify your body by boosting the circulation of lymph, the fluid that carries waste, debris, toxins, and sick cells through the lymph vessels and nodes.

Different massage techniques can range from gentle stroking to considerable pressure, include Swedish massage, lymphatic massage, sports massage, and trigger point massage, to name a few. All types move lymph through the system, but while you are cleansing, lymphatic massage is the most effective. It uses a specific degree of pressure and rhythmic circular movements to encourage lymph to move toward the heart, stimulating its circulation to clear toxins.

Another way to enhance detoxification is with acupuncture. If your intestinal tract is sluggish, for example, acupuncture can target that part of your body and speed up elimination. Likewise, it can target your lymphatic or another system that needs a push in the right direction. Acupuncture's other benefit is that it helps you deal with such initial detoxing side effects as headaches, fatigue, irritability, and even flu-like symptoms, all of which are proof that your body is cleansing itself. Acupuncture can reduce such symptoms, making detoxification easier and more pleasant.

Booster #6: Detox with Skin Brushing

Skin brushing is an easy, inexpensive, and effective practice to help eliminate toxins. Your skin is always scaling off dead cells, but you want to speed the process during a cleanse to prevent dead skin from blocking your pores. Use a soft, natural-bristle brush with a long handle—you can find them in health food stores and some pharmacies—to gently "scrub" your dry skin, from your feet and hands and towards your heart. A loofah does the job too. If possible, do this daily for several minutes. Be gentle on thinner-skinned areas such as your torso and use more pressure in thicker-skinned areas such as your back and the soles of your feet. In addition to removing dead skin cells, you are stimulating the all-important lymphatic system. For best results follow your scrub with a hot-cold plunge or shower. If you need to moisturize your skin afterward, use sesame, coconut, or other natural herbal oil instead of a drugstore product filled with toxic chemicals.

WHEN THINGS DON'T GO AS WELL AS EXPECTED

A common reason that people may start feeling worse during a detox program is undetected parasites. They were happy sharing your sugar and gluten, but once you starve them by eliminating their favorite foods and attack them with herbs, they may act out and flare up. This may show up as a rash or any of many skin problems, bloating, or diarrhea. Most conventional doctors look for parasites only when symptoms are severe. I have found parasites in many patients who had no idea or suspicion they had them, and only after something went apparently wrong during their detox program. If the program is not going well at all, you may want to stop and see a Functional Medicine doctor. Other problems that may seemingly worsen during a detox program are heavy metal toxicity, gallstones, and gout,

among others. Here are good places to look for a good practitioner in your area who knows how to deal with what you are
going through: www.functionalmedicine.org and www.ayurve-
danama.site-ym.com.

Day 6 of CLEAN7

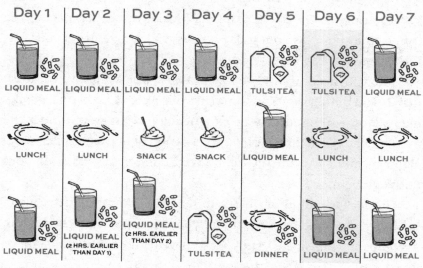

A liquid meal can be a shake, a smoothie, or a soup.

You are probably feeling better on day 6 than you have in a long
time. Most people find that hunger and food cravings are greatly
reduced by now, along with headaches, bad dreams, mood swings,
constipation, low energy, and/or the jitters. What a great feeling!

After your first solid food dinner this week, you may have noticed that your sleep was affected. Today you will have an opportunity to recover from that solid dinner (which in the context of
CLEAN7 is an indulgence), especially if you ate a little extra because
you didn't have breakfast earlier that day. It's also as a test example

of what you can do as you move forward with your life. If you have a large dinner one night, you can always make up for it by not having breakfast the next day. Doing this deliberately on days 5 and 6 should help free you from the fallacy that if you skip breakfast, your day is doomed. The CLEAN7 program frees you from the tyranny of having to eat breakfast every day. Skipping breakfast is actually a great thing to do regularly or occasionally. By lunchtime you will feel considerably better.

Now it is time to slowly go back to the eating schedule you followed on day 1. On day 5, skipping breakfast was just part of the twenty-four-hour fast, but today it's a way to recover from your first solid dinner in five days.

Today, instead of a shake for breakfast, you will have tulsi tea, just as you did on day 5, along with your Ayurvedic herbal supplements. You will essentially be experiencing a fast from dinner the evening of day 5 to lunch on day 6, a period of between sixteen and eighteen hours. At lunch, you'll have a solid meal following your dosha guidelines.

Dinner is a liquid meal. Try to have it earlier rather than later to stretch the time between it and your breakfast shake tomorrow. Accompany your shake with your Ayurvedic herbal supplements as usual. And again, if you are journaling, be sure to note your feelings and thoughts about skipping breakfast, extending the interval between meals, and the detox boosters you engaged in today.

Booster #7: Rest and Sleep

One of the biggest health challenges we face as a culture is the lack of sufficient sleep, which is when the body's important repair work is mostly done, including the work of detoxification. According to a 2016 study published in the Centers for Disease Control and Prevention's (CDC) Morbidity and Mortality Weekly Report, more than a third of American adults regularly get less than seven hours of sleep a night. Such a habit is associated with a number of chronic conditions that include diabetes, hypertension, and heart disease, as well as obesity. Lack of sufficient sleep plays a role in weight gain by creating an imbalance of the hormones that control appetite. CLEAN7 is an opportunity to start to rectify this sleep deficit. Energy levels fluctuate frequently during any detoxification program. In the first couple of days, you may feel more tired and/or get tired earlier than usual. Use this signal as an opportunity to tuck in earlier and/or sleep later than usual. (This is another good reason to start CLEAN7 on a weekend.) After a few days on the program, you may experience a natural correction of fatigue and find yourself rising earlier without being tired or not wanting to hang out in bed any longer. Adequate rest is a priority, so treat yourself gently.

Day 7 of CLEAN7

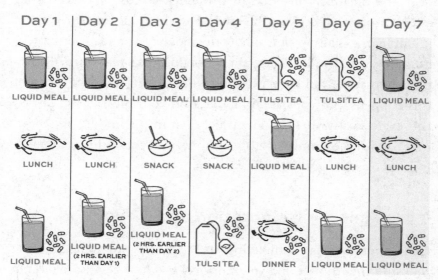

*A liquid meal can be a shake, a smoothie, or a soup.

This is your last day on CLEAN7. Or is it? Many people have such a good experience on the program that they decide to continue for another week or two, as we'll discuss in chapter 7. Day 7 is identical to day 1. By now you know the mealtime drill. Enjoy your breakfast shake, following the same guidelines you have adhered to all along, accompanied by your Ayurvedic herbal supplements. Have a solid food meal for lunch. If possible, have your dinner shake relatively early, along with your herbal supplements, to maximize the time without eating before breakfast tomorrow. Feel free to have tulsi or another herbal tea after dinner.

Booster #8: Detox with Mindful Breathing

Breathing doesn't just bring oxygen in; it is also a crucial method for releasing toxins. When you exhale carbon dioxide, you are ridding the blood of acidity in the form of carbonic acid. A simple exercise involves being mindful of your breath for a few minutes. Begin by breathing in and out through the nose and keep your attention focused on your breath. Be aware at all times if you are inhaling or exhaling. Notice how the moment you take your attention away from your breath, the autopilot kicks in—you will continue to breathe, but your attention will be elsewhere. The moment this happens, put your attention back on your breath. You can do this exercise anywhere, at any time, even in the middle of a meeting. You will be simultaneously cleaning out your lungs and quieting and clearing your mind.

Time for Celebration and Reflection

Congratulations on completing the CLEAN7 program. You just took an inner shower and you must feel and look clean. Hold on to this feeling. Remember it vividly.

By the time you complete day 7, you're going to feel significantly better overall, as well as more awake, energetic, and alert.

Some people claim they feel a natural high. Give yourself a high five! You are also going to experience a tremendous sense of accomplishment. You decided to do something different and difficult, and you managed to do it. For some of you it may even have been surprisingly easy. You may or may not have lost weight—the scale is not an accurate measure of results—but I can almost guarantee that you will have lost some volume as you can tell by how your clothes feel, particularly those jeans that were a tad too snug a week ago. Take a look at that photo of yourself before you began the program. Now take a photo of yourself after seven days, and compare the two. Your tummy will be flatter and any bloating will be significantly reduced. Your skin has a new glow and your hair is softer and shinier. You will be sleeping better, your mind will be clearer, you will feel more energy, and your body odor will be less than before, even after you've worked up a sweat exercising. And believe it or not, your poop won't be as smelly! Note all these changes in your CLEAN7 journal.

Then there are the emotional and mental results. You probably feel calmer and are enjoying a renewed mental clarity. You have demonstrated that you have the ability to take control and commit to and stick to achieving a difficult goal. You have every right to be proud, even joyful at your resolve and your success, but most of all at how you feel: Clean! It's a great feeling.

If you started CLEAN7 last Saturday, you can celebrate over the weekend, perhaps getting together with friends for a hike, a picnic, or another activity. On the other hand, you could also celebrate your success in completing one week by committing to another week on the program. Whatever you decide, don't just let tomorrow happen. Envision how you want the day to be and give it the same resolve you have demonstrated over the last week. This could manifest as taking some of the lessons you learned on CLEAN7 forward. Perhaps eliminating caffeine and/or alcohol for the week made you realize how little you need or even want either or both of them. Or maybe that nightly bowl of ice cream you used to look forward to after dinner is no longer so compelling. After completing CLEAN7 many people keep on reshaping their habits, such as skipping breakfasts or having their main meal in the middle of the day and a light dinner in the evening in order to maximize time for detoxification and enhance the quality of their sleep.

Practices Can Become Habits

In a very short time, you have built a toolkit of practices, such as the following, that you can continue to use going forward:

- Extend the interval between the last meal of one day and breakfast the next day.

- Replace dinner with tulsi tea or another herbal tea.

- Skip breakfast.

- Substitute a nutritious snack for lunch.

- Eat dinner earlier than you usually do.

- Eat breakfast later than you usually do

- Fast intermittently for twenty-four hours, by skipping both dinner and breakfast with a night's sleep in between.

You now have a whole portfolio of healthy habits to incorporate to keep toxins at bay, as well as to boost the detox processes. I encourage you to see CLEAN7 as an entry point and as something you do periodically for maintenance, just as you would maintain your car or your heating system.

Now that you cleaned your own body, keep reading. In chapter 5

I will tell you what I learned about how to detox my mind, and in chapter 6 how I joined a movement to clean the planet that complements my work of helping people get clean. Finally, in chapter 7, I will tell you different ways you can go from here to make the experience you just had a life-lasting one.

5

Detox Your Mind by Becoming Present

Of all the symptoms that I was experiencing when I got sick during my years of training in New York, the scariest one was in my mind. The constant repetitive stream of negative thoughts was draining my vital energy as it prevented me from functioning and paralyzed me from even trying to get better. From the moment I woke up until I fell asleep, there were constant thoughts in my mind. Often I couldn't sleep, because I could not turn them off. They were mostly negative. Some of them scary. Self-judging, self-deprecating, exhausting. I didn't have a single class in medical school that gave me the tools to even think about this problem, let alone understand it. Psychiatry was more concerned with how chemicals can alter the course of mental disorders. But that is not what I was trying to understand. I am not talking about serious mental health issues such as bipolar disorder and schizophrenia. I am talking about the pervasive unease that most people experience from a mind that cannot seem to stop blaming them, judging them, and tainting any other experience they may have while this automatic negative stream of thoughts is going on.

Initially, I had so many thoughts whirling through my mind that I thought I was going mad. I even had full conversations going on in my head. At the time, there was a doctor at Lenox Hill Hospital with whom I did not get along. No one did. He was the chief of the cardiac catheterization lab. He was rude and verbally abusive. He got away with it because his department was the biggest moneymaker for the hospital. I found myself having arguments in my mind with him, in which I told him what I thought about him and he would scream at me—all in my head. I was in the subway one morning on my way to work, having one of my mental fights with this guy, when I saw someone who was talking to himself out loud. He seemed as if he had gone mad. He was having arguments with imaginary people, just as I was, but he was doing it out loud. A sense of panic invaded me as these thoughts appeared in my mind: "That is me. That is exactly what is happening to me. Am I going to start doing it out loud next? Why can't I stop these thoughts? Why can't I think of better thoughts? But wait, I am not choosing these thoughts. They just appear on their own. And if I am not choosing my thoughts, who is?"

The one thing that was clear to me was that these were not just thoughts that came and went. They grabbed my attention. And once I was deep into them, they changed my body chemistry in a bad way. During the fights in my head my heart would start racing and my muscles got tense. My adrenalin was pumping almost as much as it would if I were getting into an actual physical fight. My blood pressure went up and I got so lost in thought that I got distracted when walking around, sometimes bumping into people on the streets or almost getting run over by a cab. This is known as the fight-or-flight reaction. In my case, my body was getting ready to fight. But there was no one there. It was all in my mind.

The fight-or-flight reaction is a survival mechanism that is part of most animals' basic design. It allows escaping or confronting a predator. If one of our ancient ancestors was suddenly attacked and chased by a tiger, that survival mechanism would maximize the chances of escape. Once our ancestors managed to escape and the tiger went away, the fight-or-flight reaction would disappear, and things would go back to normal. But there is a glitch in our design. Even if the danger is not actually there, if you just think about it, the fight-or-flight reaction gets triggered. I was being chased by a tiger in my mind—all the time. My fight-or-flight reaction was my constant state. This realization scared me. The thought, "I am mad," kept on popping into my mind. "I need help," I decided.

The psychiatrist I saw wanted to start me on medications, but I did not want to spend my life on pills. I wanted to understand what was wrong with me. So I started to read. At first, I looked in books on psychiatry. There were lots of classifications of mental disorders, but none of them answered my questions: "Who is choosing my thoughts and how can I stop them?" Every now and then I found a quote by someone that made sense to me and I would read more of that author's work. Soon I ended up in the self-help and new-age sections of the bookstore, where I found some interesting books. One of them was Shakti Gawain's book, *Creative Visualization*. The basic premise is that if you imagine something you want very vividly, in great detail, it will manifest in your life. Abraham and Esther Hicks's book, *The Law of Attraction*, is also great. It states that the universe will bring you whatever it is that you spend time desiring and visualizing. I delved into quantum physics as the framework of thinking that explained these phenomena. We are all made of energy. Energy attracts energy of the same frequency of vibration. What you think is what you become. It all made sense. But it didn't really help me. I found myself following their instructions, setting up my space, and taking time to visualize. But as soon as I started, I noticed my negative thoughts got even louder.

The more I read and observed everybody around me, the more it became clear that I was not the only one having this experience with thoughts. Many people were. I started observing that some people had streams of thoughts that forced their attention into their heads, even while having a conversation with me. They were half there and half in their heads. Once I saw that in myself, I started to see it in others as well. Their stares became empty. If I suddenly stopped talking or mumbled something unintelligible, they wouldn't immediately notice. They were not "present." Often, neither was I.

As I kept reading and looking for answers, I also went to counselors and therapists. They were all somewhat helpful, even if only because they listened to me. But not one of them helped me understand my predicament any better. One therapist was big into "positive thinking." He told me that I could train my mind to change the negative thoughts for positive ones. "Think positive" was his mantra. But this is easier said than done. I tried hard. The moment I became aware that I was in the middle of one of my mental movies that triggered my fight-or-flight response, I threw in positive thoughts. I did this again and again and again. In time, I was able to replace the negative thoughts with positive ones, for a short while. And then, like an elastic band that has been stretched to the max, the moment I got distracted, the band recoiled and the negative thoughts snapped back with a vengeance. At least this exercise gave me hope that I could momentarily choose my thoughts. The negative ones popped up by themselves. If I had a choice, I wouldn't be thinking them. But the positive ones I did choose myself. It took effort to keep the awareness that my mind was just thinking thoughts on its own and even more effort to come up with positive thoughts and keep them going. It was exhausting. I noticed that some people think positively most of the time. Most of the ones I asked couldn't really explain to me how I could do it myself. It was as if they were just born with it. For me, trying to "think positive" was exhausting.

It was around this time that I decided to get back into physical shape, since I had gained so much weight from all the years of hospital food and stress. I started lifting weights and got into running, which I enjoyed enormously. I learned a breathing technique that allowed me to run for much longer than I thought I could. As I ran, I consciously took a breath with each step, two breaths in and two breaths out, each breath timed exactly to each step (breathe in when your right foot goes to the front and, without exhaling, again when your left foot goes to the front; the two in are through the nose, the two out are through the mouth). I breathed in through my nose and breathed out my mouth. After a few minutes I entered a trance-like state. My thoughts started waning in strength and quantity. The more I put my attention on synchronizing my breath with each step, the fewer thoughts appeared, until there were no thoughts at all. I became the running. Breath, muscles, rhythm, and nothing else. I remembered that this was the same state I achieved years earlier in Uruguay when I was training and competing in tae kwon do. It gave me a great sense of freedom. After running, sometimes for two hours, I felt more rested and energized than before I started. I just wanted to run all day long. I became addicted to running. I was dependent on it for my sanity. I thought I had found the solution—until I sprained my ankle one day, and within a few days of not running, I was back where I started: inner hell.

I shared what I had learned through running with one of my therapists. He gave me a book that really helped: *Flow* by Mihaly Csikszentmihalyi. The state of flow is that thoughtless state (free of any thoughts, negative or positive) that people enter when they are so focused in the present that there is no space left in the mind for anything else, including thoughts. Athletes experience this state when training and competing, as do dancers when dancing, surfers when surfing, musicians when playing their instrument, actors when acting, surgeons when operating. Whatever experience you are having when you enter the state of Flow will be enjoyed and

remembered vividly. Sometimes the state of Flow is entered accidentally, when in great danger for example. In this state people
are capable of pretty unbelievable things. It is likely in part due to
the fight-or-flight hormones, but when in Flow, they get stronger.
An example is a mother lifting up a car to rescue her child from
beneath it. We've all heard about or witnessed something like that.
Some people do really dangerous things that require them to enter
that state as a matter of survival. If you start arguing with your boss
in your head while skydiving, you may end up dead. I believe that
people always, knowingly or unknowingly, intentionally seek that
state. They also enjoy watching or being in the presence of others
who are in that state. Professional athletes, dancers, surfers, actors
and anyone else who performs at high levels enter the state of presence, which is part of their appeal.

The book *Flow* helped me grasp the concept of what being present actually means and how it explains why people who enter the
state of flow are more often happier and healthier than those who
never or rarely do. But if I couldn't run, I couldn't enter this state.
There had to be another way.

One day, hunting for some book references, I found myself in
the Eastern philosophy section of the bookstore. A book literally
fell in my hands and opened up to a page titled "Meditation." In
it, meditation was described as a practice that can help slow down
the stream of repetitive automatic thoughts and eventually stop
them. The mind, constantly jumping from thought to thought was
compared to a monkey jumping nonstop from branch to branch,
or to a hungry dog that obstinately gnaws on a bone, just as the
mind chews on certain thoughts. I bought a bunch of books on
meditation and started following their instructions. Find a quiet
place, sit with your back straight, close your eyes, and take a few
deep breaths. Before I could take the next step, I noticed that my
thoughts seemed to increase and get stronger. I felt I just could not
do it. That meditation wasn't for me.

One day, my friend Fernando said he would take me to a school of meditation. We drove north in New York State and arrived at a beautiful set of buildings in the middle of some gorgeous gardens. "Come," he said, "the meditation intensive is starting." I followed him into a big conference room where hundreds of people were sitting on the floor, chanting. I later found out that this was a special day, the day of the teacher. After a while, the meditation teacher came into the hall and joined the chanting. There was something incredibly special about her, an intense glow. She had the strongest magnetism of anyone I had ever encountered. That is when it hit me that she was fully present. As the chanting went on I became fascinated by her every movement, which was as if in slow motion. I had never seen anyone move in that way. I am not sure how long I stayed there, but after a while I felt somewhat lightheaded, so I went outside.

I must have looked stressed because a meditation student assigned as my host came out to ask me if I was okay. I said that I was dizzy, but fine. She asked me to follow her so we could find a place to sit down. As we were walking down a corridor, a door opened and the meditation teacher stepped out, almost bumping into us. "Hi, Prema," she greeted my host. "And what is your name?" she asked me. "My name is Alejandro," I replied. "What do you do, Alejandro?"' she asked. "I am a doctor," I replied. "What kind?" "A cardiologist." "Oh, the heart," she said, bursting into laughter and slapped my chest, right over my heart. What happened next is impossible to describe accurately, but I'll give it a try. There was no experience of me being inside a body looking out through my eyes. I was everywhere. I was everything. There was no space and time. Initially my feeling was one of fear, but soon it transformed into the most amazing feeling of happiness I had ever experienced. It went beyond happiness. It was peace.

It wasn't me experiencing something. There was no difference between the experience and the experiencer. There was not a single thought in my mind. I am not sure how long I remained in that state; it must have been a few minutes, but it seemed eternal. I have been searching for a way to enter that state ever since—and stay there. I have had a few flashes of it since. All of them happened in the most unexpected moments and never during any meditation technique or practice.

Today I understand that state is our natural state, our birthright. It is the state of pure presence, which is what I think of as enlightenment. Because of the unnatural way in which we live, soon after we are born we are trained to put our attention into thought, into an identity. We start defining who we are, what we like, and what we don't like. But we are always, often without knowing it, somehow looking to return to that state of pure presence. We play sports, we dance, we do dangerous activities, we pray, we make love, we eat, we do whatever it is, in part, to experience it again.

A big part of why negative thoughts keep repeating is the accumulation of ama, which I described in chapter 3. Ama is the accumulation of toxic molecules (endogenous and exogenous) and the mucus and fat that the body generates and retains to defend itself from them. This physical ama has a low vibrational frequency and by resonance attracts and amplifies thoughts and emotions of a similar vibrational frequency, the quantum ama. And vice versa.

As we enter and go through the CLEAN7 program, toxic chemicals will be neutralized, made water soluble, and eliminated and so will the mucus and fat that were serving the purpose of buffering the irritation these toxic molecules cause. This will create an inner condition with less of a hold on quantum ama. This is why nightmares and mood swings can occur while on the program. But this is also the perfect time to learn and practice some version of meditation, since it will not only be facilitated by the elimination of physical ama, but it will in turn also boost its elimination.

There is no argument about the value of meditation for well-being. There are plenty of scientific studies that prove the benefits.

But people get intimidated even by the word *meditation* itself. It seems so unattainable that people don't even try it. That is why I am giving you three simple exercises that work and are easy to do. They take only a few minutes a day. These are not to "replace" longer meditation practices. Rather, they are to get you started. And even if you already are an experienced meditator, these exercises will enhance your meditation practice. During CLEAN7, I encourage you to use one of these three techniques for "becoming present," or all of them, for seven minutes every day. They will make your "presence muscle" stronger.

The Anchor

At any time of the day, take seven minutes to anchor your attention in the present. To do so, you will direct your attention fully into places that are always in the present—your body, your breath, whatever you see and hear around you. Sit in a chair with your back straight. Keep your eyes open. Rest the palms of your hands comfortably on your thighs. Take a deep breath and exhale slowly. Start by putting your attention in your body. Feel your feet from inside, your calves, your knees, your bottom and back against the chair, your abdomen, arms, hands, and head. Feel your body intensely from inside. Be mindful not to tense your muscles; instead keep them relaxed, but feel your body, all of it at the same time, all the time. If thoughts appear, don't fight them. Don't try to stop them, just let them be and continue to focus your attention on feeling your body intensely from inside, this will most likely happen for the whole seven minutes. Thoughts will appear. They may even steal your attention, but if you stay vigilant, you will soon catch yourself getting lost in thought. When you do, don't judge yourself or think you have failed to do the exercise correctly. Just go back to feeling your body. Once you are doing that, also put some attention on your breath. Keep feeling your body, but also pay attention to your breath. Whether your breath is on autopilot or you are consciously and voluntarily breathing in and out doesn't matter. What matters is that at all times you know if you are breathing in or out, at the same time as you are feeling your body from the inside. Once you are feeling your body and noticing your breath, put some of your attention in what you see and hear all around you, without moving your eyes. Just notice whatever falls in your field of vision, and whatever sounds are happening moment to moment. That's it. Do that for seven minutes every day. If you can do it more than once, fantastic. If you skip it one day, do it the next.

When your attention is flowing into anything in the present, there will be less attention left to flow into thought. As long as you are feeling your body, noticing your breath going in and out, seeing, and listening, your attention is anchored in the present and negative thoughts become weaker. When practiced consistently, you will strengthen your ability to direct most of your attention into your body, breath, and surroundings. You may even enter the state of flow, in which all your attention is on your body and breath and you become fully present.

The Anchor in Motion

The meditation technique above has something in common with most of the meditation techniques that I learned during my search: they are all done by stopping everything else that you are doing. You make some time, you sit down, usually in an empty quiet room, and you go inside. And then you stand up and go on with your busy life. This will also gradually percolate into your daily life and it will have a positive effect. You will be calmer. You will become a better listener. You will stop yourself getting lost in thought. But there is also something you can do to lessen the grip of unwanted thoughts during your active hours. This may sound strange but it works and I urge you to try it out a few times. At any moment during the day, whether you are in a meeting at work or talking and playing with your kids, put some of your attention in your feet. Feel your feet from inside. Feel the temperature, the humidity, feel your feet touching your shoes, pressing against the floor. Don't just do it for an instant. Keep doing it. Keep doing whatever you are doing and at the same time, continue to feel your feet from inside. It may seem counterintuitive to do that in the middle of doing other things. You may fear that by putting some attention on your feet you will be stealing attention from thinking about what you are going to say next, or from understanding what someone is telling you. But this is not what happens. Even if you are not fully aware, regardless of whatever else you are doing, there are thoughts happening involuntarily, stealing your attention. That is why so many people seem absent at times even in the middle of an important discussion. But even if automatic thoughts don't completely steal you from the present, there is an ongoing background noise made of thoughts. Sometimes they are hard to detect because we experience them as our normal "interpreting and measuring" self. They are thoughts that tell you something about what is happening, such as, "This is interesting," "He is lying," or "I can't believe she is saying that." Or you are guessing in your head what the other person is going to say. Or making mental notes of things that you have to do next. We experience these thoughts as us. We don't know anything different. We never questioned it before. When you direct some of that attention into the present you will become mentally clearer, allowing more space for connection and creativity to occur. Whatever you need to say will flow out in a more eloquent manner than usual. Because at the moment you are speaking or listening you will also have some attention in your feet, which are in the present, you will become more present yourself. Everyone in the work meeting will notice that, you will command their attention, and the meeting will go better than you expected. If you are with your kids, you will see that they respond to you differently. You will be more present, which they will feel as love.

The Ruskin School of Acting
Repetition Exercise

This exercise is a foundation exercise that was taught by Sanford Meisner (1905–1997) in his acting technique classes, and it continues to be the first piece of the work taught at the Ruskin School in Los Angeles, California, and by any authorized Meisner teacher. John Ruskin was Sanford Meisner's apprentice and taught with him at the Neighborhood Playhouse in New York City before opening the Ruskin School of Acting in Los Angeles. The exercise is designed to eliminate intellectuality from the actor's instrument, stop you from thinking, and teach you to put all your focus on your partner. The brilliance of this exercise is that in doing it, you are brought entirely into the present moment. And because there is nothing to think about other than what you see in your partner's behavior, from one second to the next, you are forced to be entirely in the moment. Over many years of teaching it, my good friend John Ruskin came to understand that this exercise isn't just something that can help actors. Non-actors, people in recovery, mothers, fathers, businesspeople, his own children, and others would benefit by doing it because it is the fastest way to get out of your head and into your heart. John thought it would help my patients. Meisner would say you're either in your head or your heart, that they are mutually exclusive, and that's true. To be able to turn off the incessant voices in your head is such a gift and this very simple exercise gets you there.

As with any exercise, it takes a little practice, so we'll go in stages. First, get comfortable with the exercise and then it can become deeper and more powerful.

You have probably had the experience of doing a good deed or being in the middle of helping a friend, when your focus and attention is fully on someone outside of yourself, and your mind quiets. The voices slow down and even stop. This repetition exercise is founded on the same principle. You will need a partner to do this exercise.

Step 1: External Details

Sit or stand across from your partner. The first time you try this exercise, decide who will go first. That person looks at the other person and very simply says what he or she sees. For example, if you are the initiator and your partner is wearing a blue shirt, then you might simply say, "Blue shirt." The partner should then repeat, "Blue shirt," exactly as heard, with complete attention on you and nothing to think about. The partner should resist any desire to be clever or make "Blue shirt" sound different. Then you put all your focus on how your partner says, "Blue shirt" and try to repeat it the exact same way, almost like a robot. Continue to repeat "Blue shirt" back and forth, very simply, without trying to make it different, until there is something else you notice about your partner perhaps, "Brown eyes." Say that new phrase and then you and your partner repeat it back and forth until the next observation, such as "Glasses," "Blond hair," etc. Continue to repeat the new word back and forth until you see the next thing and so on and so forth with one person continuing to initiate the change in words.

After a few minutes, switch, so your partner becomes the initiator. Once you've gotten the hang of this flow, either partner can initiate the change in repetition, changing the new word as inspired, based on saying what each sees in or on the other.

Step 2: Physical Behavior

Once you are used to noticing external things about your partner, you're ready to move to the next step, which is reading physical behavior. Behavior is the physical movements people make, such as "looking away," "fidgeting," "swaying," "laughing," etc. Add those words to your observations.

Step 3: Emotional Behavior

This is where you begin to say what you believe your partner is experiencing inside. Emotions manifest as behavior and we are learning to read behavior. So, if you see your partner look away, then say "looked away." If he or she appears shy, distracted, uncomfortable, happy, sad, embarrassed, etc., then say that. But keep the words simple—by simply using any of those very words if they apply. Now it is very important to remember that you're just taking your best guess from observing them, not accusing or manipulating the person, but rather saying what you see in them. The partner should be able at this point to repeat that statement, "You're shy," without thinking, and yet the instinctive response will let you know if you're right or wrong. It's not about being right, it's about really searching, keeping your focus on the other person and moving from one moment to the next without thinking. It doesn't matter whether you are right or wrong. All that matters is that you use the word repetition to keep you mindlessly repeating and staying in contact with your partner.

You aren't trying to make anything happen here! If you're trying to be clever, you're still in your head. If you're thinking about what to say next, don't. Just put 100 percent of your attention on your partner, repeat what you hear, and without thinking, pick up the next piece of behavior that you see in your partner and just say it! Whenever you get distracted or mixed up, take a deep breath, put all your focus back onto your partner, and repeat the words. That's what keeps you present, in the moment, and connected to your partner.

Sandy Meisner always said, "Act before you think" and in this part of the work, this is your goal: "Repeat before you think."

The purpose of the repetition exercise is very simple—to stop you from thinking and teach you to put your focus completely on your partner's behavior.

My friend John has practiced meditation since he was thirteen years old to try to quiet his busy mind and thoughts. When he found Sandy Meisner and the Meisner Technique, he discovered a way to get to that place of thoughtlessness more immediately and has been practicing it now for thirty-five years. Meisner invented it to train actors to be present and in their heart onstage or in front of the camera, but it was so beyond that in its practice. It was so universal in helping everyone stop thinking so much and allow themselves to be more present in the moment with themselves and others. It deepens and after much practice it begins to sound like human dialogue where each moment changes as you get more masterful at picking up your partner's behavior and naming it in the repetition exercise.

Personally, these exercises have been a lifesaver. The first two I do all the time. The third one, or a version of it, I do sometimes. Training the muscle of presence is like training any muscle. You exercise it, it gets stronger. They have helped me in every aspect of my life. CLEAN7 is a great time to put them to the test and see for yourself. If impressed, you can adopt them long term. For more info on John's work visit www.ruskinschool.com.

6

As Above, So Below: CLEAN Meets ORGANIC INDIA

There are many meanings to the phrase "As above, so below." A spiritual teacher could say it means that life on Earth can be as it is in heaven. A physicist could be talking about how an atom is very much like the solar system, its nucleus like the sun and the electrons orbiting around it like the different planets. To me, as a doctor seeking for solutions in nature, it means that the planet Earth is a living organism much like the human body: Its rivers are like arteries, its forests are like lungs, and we humans are like one of the many types of cells circulating within it. I see humans as the red blood cells of the planet. And because we are cells in this planetary body, detoxification of the human body alone is not enough. Would you remove and clean the fish in your fish tank and then throw them back into the tank's dirty water? The planet is our fish tank. Do you want to live your life swimming in dirty water? How do we clean our tank?

Synchronicities

About ten years ago, my friend Steven was traveling around India on business. One morning, on a plane from Delhi to Lucknow, he saw a man dressed in a white kurta who seemed so happy and at ease that Steven wondered what his deal was. After a day of meetings Steven went to catch his return flight to Delhi. In the lounge, waiting to board Steven's flight, was the same man he had seen that morning. Steven went up to him, introduced himself and flat out asked him: "What do you do? What do you eat? You seem so happy; I want to do what you do."

The man responded that his name is Bharat Mitra. He had just spent the day in Lucknow, where he had organized a big conference for medical doctors to teach them about wellness, holistic medicine, and Ayurvedic herbs. Then out of the blue Bharat said, "Next year I want to bring a doctor from America to the conference whose book, *CLEAN*, really resonates with me. His name is Alejandro Junger." "Synchronicity!" Steven said, "He is like my brother," and immediately called me and put me on the phone with Bharat. We hit it off right away and made plans to meet in person a few days later, since we were both going to be in Australia. Another synchronicity.

I met Bharat and his wife, Bhavani, at their home in Byron Bay, Australia, and had the same first impression as Steven. Both radiated health and happiness. Their story blew my mind. They had not only figured out *how* to clean the tank, they were doing it. They were doing for the planetary body what I was doing for the individual human bodies circulating within it. We couldn't stop talking. We told each other our life stories.

A Command Becomes Reality,
How ORGANIC INDIA Was Born

Bharat left his native Israel at age seventeen seeking enlightenment. His search eventually took him to Lucknow where he found his guru, Papaji. Bhavani had also gone to India in her spiritual search and became a student of Papaji. That is where Bharat and Bhavani met, fell in love, and got married. Most gurus are monks or swamis, but Papaji was a householder. He taught and guided people to experience enlightenment in their everyday lives without having to renounce the world.

Bharat recalls, "I was totally dedicated to Papaji and to spiritual truth. I never had any interest whatsoever in anything worldly." But in 1996, about a year before he passed away, Papaji told Bharat, "Start a private limited company." "Yes, Papaji," he dutifully replied, but when his guru left the room he turned to a friend and asked, "What's a private limited company?" The friend explained that it was a commercial entity. Papaji's only comment was, "This company will help everybody!" Bharat Mitra didn't know what the company would do. He told me, "The one thing I knew in my heart was that the core purpose of this company was to be a vehicle of consciousness, by being a living embodiment of love in action."

At that time, India was opening itself to international business. Bharat and Bhavani began the business by trading goods from and to India. They started with many different items produced in India such as rugs and handcrafts. After spending countless hours in an office and closing many trading deals, Bharat had a strong gut feeling that this company was going to grow globally. He ran to Papaji's house, prostrated himself at his feet, and said, "Papaji, please. I don't want any of it. All I ever wanted is to serve you. Please take it away."

Papaji looked at him with a big smile on his face and said, "But that's why you must do it. Because you don't want anything, that's why it can happen." This is how ORGANIC INDIA was born.

From Rugs to Herbs

During many years with Papaji, Bharat and Bhavani had witnessed firsthand the healing power of Ayurvedic Medicine, particularly using Ayurvedic herbs. Bharat told me about a man with leukemia, who after failing strong chemotherapy, was told he had two or three weeks to live and was sent home to die. His wife asked him what he wanted to do in his last few weeks of life. The man replied, "I want to see Papaji." The couple withdrew all their savings from the bank and Bharat arranged for an ambulance airplane to transport them from Delhi to Lucknow, complete with oxygen tanks. When they arrived at Papaji's house and told him that the man had been given two weeks to live, Papaji replied, "Nobody can decide when you die," and sent him to see an Ayurvedic doctor who treated him with herbs and dosha-specific dietary guidelines. Eight months later, the man and his wife left Lucknow healthy and laughing. Bharat recalls that he was still alive and well at least five years later.

This and other examples of the healing, restorative, and life-enhancing powers of Ayurvedic Medicine, especially Ayurvedic herbs, motivated Bharat and Bhavani to find herbal and other Ayurvedic Medicines and supplements for all the people who were coming to Lucknow to see Papaji and for trading internationally. Bharat Mitra searched the whole country looking for sources of good quality Ayurvedic herbs. Shockingly, all the sources of herbs he could find were of very poor quality and were kept in dusty, unhygienic storerooms (called "go-downs" in India). Even worse, ever since the so-called green revolution in India, the massive amounts of modern chemical fertilizers, pesticides, and herbicides had resulted in toxic crops, clearly unusable as herbal medicines or supplements. It became clear that Ayurvedic herbs must be grown organically. It also became clear that farming chemicals are toxic not only when you consume them, but also affect everything related to them.

Dry Land, Deep Pain

Bharat explained to me that initially the modern farming chemicals produced a higher yield of crops, so farmers got hooked. However, they found that after a few years the land needed more and more agricultural chemicals to maintain the same yield. The chemicals were expensive and so were the seeds designed to survive the chemical attack. The farmers' bank accounts were drying up and so was their land, which had become dependent on more chemicals. Having no other resources, the farmers needed to mortgage their land to pay for the seeds and chemicals, in the hope that they would get a crop they could sell. This resulted in many farmers losing their land, losing their ability to provide for their families, and losing their dignity, which was unbearable for them. Sad beyond words, many of these farmers saw that the only way out of this deplorable situation was to commit suicide. Bharat found out that 12,000 to 19,000 farmers were committing suicide every year. Bharat and Bhavani felt compelled to do something about this and a vision for a perfect solution was born: producing organically grown Ayurvedic herbal medicines in partnership with farmers. In this way they would be able to make high-quality healing herbs available for consumers, while at the same time teaching farmers to return to organic traditional farming and free themselves from the deadly trap they were in.

Dr. Narendra Singh, Prana Whisperer

With this vision in mind Bharat started searching for advice from experts in Ayurvedic herbs. He was led to a legend in the city of Lucknow, Dr. Narendra Singh, a medical doctor who was also the president and founder of the International Institute for Herbal Medicine. For years he was the head of the pharmacological department at the prestigious King George's Medical University, conducting in-depth research in Ayurvedic medicinal herbs.

For decades, Dr. Narendra himself had looked for quality Ayurvedic herbs to give his patients and use in his clinical trials but had found none. So he took it upon himself to find the reason for that. He spoke to as many experts as he could and studied the ancient Ayurvedic textbooks, some of them in Sanskrit. After years of study he resolved the great mystery of why he was not getting the same results with herbs that he had witnessed from his teachers years before. It was because the herbs were no longer being grown and prepared in the right way. The way the seeds are planted, how much water they get, and how they are harvested, dried, mixed, and prepared for the patient are all essential to their quality. The potency of Ayurvedic herbs depends on the life force within them. Dr. Narendra explained that plants are vehicles of healing frequencies that carry nature's inherent intelligence, and they can affect cells in different ways, assisting with balance, repair, and nutrition and can even alter gene expression for the better. This life force is called *prana,* and it must be preserved, or the herbs will give you only nutrients and antioxidants, which although beneficial, are but a small part of the power of herbs.

Herbs carry the intelligence of nature and cause different effects depending on their conditions. Ashwagandha, for example, will tone up a tired adrenal gland if exhaustion is the condition but will tone it down if stress is predominant. Because it helps the body adapt, it is known as an adaptogen. Dr. Narendra created his own herbal gardens following the strict standards and conditions his research had uncovered and started treating his patients with them. He was amazed at the results. And his legendary status grew.

Bharat visited Dr. Narendra's office to witness the results with patients and to see the gardens. Bharat was so impressed he told Dr. Narendra that ORGANIC INDIA wanted to scale up the cultivation of his herbs and make them available to the world. Narendra said it was impossible to do it as a business and that he was not interested in profiting from such an endeavor. He had never even charged a single patient in decades. "It just can't be done," he declared. "Why?" asked Bharat. "Because even if we figured out how to scale up what I do in my gardens, no farmer would be crazy enough to start planting something that, if not sold, they cannot eat themselves or sell to someone else. It's too risky. I come from a village of farmers. I know how they think and feel," responded Narendra forcefully.

But Bharat would not give up. He visited Narendra whenever he could and got him to start thinking big. "You cannot retire to your village and let this knowledge go into hiding again. This knowledge is too important," he told Narendra. "We have a responsibility to share this knowledge with humanity. If we are unable to maintain the same quality that you offer your patients while we scale up, then we will not do it at all. But we must at least explore the possibility and give it all we have." As time went by, Dr. Narendra's resistance turned into inspiration, passion, and a plan.

After months of research, trials and errors, Bharat, Bhavani, and Narendra figured out how it could be done. They created a large garden in Lucknow to test their ideas. And it worked. A deep trusting friendship developed as well, so when it was time to enroll the first farmers, Narendra took Bharat to Azamgarh, his native village. At a village meeting with the farmers, Narendra and Bharat offered the assembled farmers the opportunity to be a part of the beginning of an organic revolution in India that would benefit farmers, their families, their villages, the whole country, and the Earth itself. After explaining that the first crop would be tulsi, the mother of all healing herbs, Bharat asked, "Who wants to join in?" The silence was deafening.

Then one farmer spoke up. "We would be willing to sign on to grow rice or wheat. Everybody who comes to the village makes promises, but nobody keeps them," he said. "You say you will buy the tulsi, but I cannot eat tulsi and I cannot sell it if you don't buy it. You want me to trust you with my life. I don't have anything else. What I grow is all I have for my family and me." Bharat looked at Narendra, who smiled as if saying, "I told you so."

Bharat gave them his word that he wouldn't let them down, and mostly because of their trust and love for Dr. Narendra, the chief of the village, Kailash Nath Singh, and eight other farmers joined in. The ORGANIC INDIA team brought the seeds and the machinery, and under Dr. Narendra's guidance, taught the famers how to plant, water, harvest, dry, and prepare the tulsi. They also taught the community how to use all the bio-waste of the entire village to create organic compost to enrich the soil and increase crop yields. Collectively, preparing compost brought the entire community together.

Not surprisingly, the first harvest wasn't usable, due to the chemical residue in the soil, but ORGANIC INDIA paid the farmers as promised for the crop. The next year twenty-two more farmers joined after seeing that the original farmers had been paid. One of the farmers, who was initially the loudest opponent, changed his mind and decided to get on board. "Why?" Bharat asked him. "The birds of my childhood have returned to the fields," he replied.

Thanks to ORGANIC INDIA, whole villages have revived. The company has installed bore wells and irrigation systems, built medical clinics, supported schools, and provided women's education and well-being in these villages. The younger generation is now keen on agriculture because they realize that the more effort they put in, the more they will get back. The villagers have not just an income, but also a sustainable environment; good health for themselves, their families, and their livestock; and very importantly, their dignity and pride in providing home, health, and happiness for their families and village communities.

At the first function with the farmers to celebrate after a few years of work, Bharat Mitra praised Kailash Nath Singh, citing his vision and courage to be the first farmer to join. Kailash came to the stage and said, "Thank you very much, but I didn't have vision. I didn't have courage. I was actually contemplating committing suicide. I simply did not think I had anything to lose." Years later Kailash died a happy man. He had fulfilled his function. His family still benefits from the love he had to give, which at one point was almost lost prematurely.

Today, there are thousands of farmers, all growing their crops organically, in many villages all over India, and not one has left the company in eighteen years. According to Bharat, the happiness he sees in their faces is the reason for the happiness Steven saw on his face that first time they met.

Meeting the Master

As Bharat continued his stories, he suddenly had an idea; "You need to come to Lucknow and see for yourself," he said. "Yes," I answered. When I arrived at the doctor's house four months later, there was a line of people waiting to see him that stretched around the block. Inside his office it seemed like chaos. Dr. Narendra was sitting behind a large desk piled with patients' charts and other documents. To his left were a professor of medicine at one of Lucknow's teaching hospitals and a graduate of religious studies. Both were taking notes. In front of Dr. Narendra were several of his patients—some alone, some with their family members—sitting wherever they could. He would talk to one patient, then jump to another, then another, in no apparent order. Every now and then he would snap his fingers and four young men would run to get him whatever he needed, as if deciphering the finger snap telepathically. Narendra's office was buzzing. Together with the outside traffic noise, honking, and the loud music from the temple across the street, my mind just couldn't take it all in. I sat to his right and Narendra immediately started telling me about the patients he was seeing. After two minutes everything seemed to slow down and I suddenly perceived everything differently—total order, stillness, peaceful presence.

What I witnessed blew my mind. This is what I saw and heard, from the patients themselves and from reviewing their medical charts. A man had been on dialysis for years before seeing Narendra. With some dietary advice according to Ayurvedic principles, but mostly with herbs, Narendra had helped him get his kidneys working again. When I saw the man, he had been off dialysis for a year. I saw another man whose liver had been devastated by cirrhosis and had been under Dr. Narendra's care for two years. He had brought with him his latest blood tests, which revealed normal liver function. I saw a woman whose skin had been buried in eczema, now with glowing, pink skin. The photos of her skin before treatment were unrecognizable. With patient after patient, I was witnessing people who had reversed long-standing chronic diseases that had been worsening for years.

Many of Dr. Narendra's patients had been failures of modern medicine who tried Ayurveda as their last resort. One case was very surprising. A woman who had severe arthritis to the point of needing a wheelchair most of the time was now reporting that she was even climbing stairs. It had made a huge difference in her life. She was in tears. I observed that she was very overweight. I asked Narendra what dietary prescription she had gotten. "None," he replied, "only herbs." "Why?" I asked. "Because she has little willpower, and if I gave her both herbs and dietary instructions, she would not have done either," he answered. "I had to choose. I chose herbs." "But isn't that similar to doctors that just give a pill for an ill?" I asked. "Far from it," Narendra answered. "Western medications are great and necessary in some cases. It is a good thing we have them. They mostly act by exciting or inhibiting receptors in cells that in turn trigger or prevent the cell from functioning in a certain way. Exciting or inhibiting receptors is like solving mathematics problems by adding or subtracting sticks; using herbs is like solving algebra with quantum supercomputers of the future. The prana in Ayurvedic herbs can affect receptors and much more. And I am not talking about prana as a mysterious force that acts like praying. Prana can affect cells just like a sustained high-frequency sound note can shatter glass, or X-rays can damage your genes. It is like music to your cells. And its effects go beyond cells. Herbal prana can change your emotions and your thoughts, recalibrate your intuition, and even assist your soul in its journey. That is why it is so important to conserve this vibrational frequency; you want your whole body to hear this music. It needs to be loud and in tune."

Ayur-CLEAN

Week after week I sat with Dr. Narendra in awe. He was a serious man, but when he laughed, it was as though the sun came out. One day he snapped his fingers and a copy of my first book, *CLEAN*, was immediately brought to him. He looked at me and said, "I read it. This is an Ayurvedic Medicine book." "It is more a Functional Medicine book," I argued. "Same thing," said Narendra. He then went on to explain how Functional Medicine already has many Ayurvedic principles in it and how I could add more Ayurvedic principles and herbs to make the detox program deeper, more intense, and even more beneficial. This is how CLEAN7 was born.

Dr. Narendra was incredibly knowledgeable in both Western and Ayurvedic Medicines and had a unique ability to explain how they were similar in so many ways. We had long discussions about hepatocytes (liver cells), the p450 enzymes (the main detox enzymes), the nutrients needed to support them, how prana played a role, and how the doshas affect everything. He was as passionate about detoxification as I am and not only with regard to the human body. He hammered into my brain that if there is no concomitant planetary detox as well, we are not helping this world in the long run.

Missions That Resonate, Above and Below

Cleansing and detoxification had helped me completely resolve my depression, allergies, and irritable bowel syndrome. Since then it has been the most powerful tool in my personal and medical practice toolbox. I made it my mission to spread the word and inspire more and more people to benefit from it. I wrote the book *CLEAN*, in which I laid out a twenty-one-day program with instructions for anyone to do it by preparing all their meals, both liquid and solid, from only whole foods. I also created a company, CLEAN, that provides the shakes for the liquid meals and a combination of supplements that enhances the detox process for those who have no time or interest in preparing everything on their own. My team and I have transformed thousands of lives all over the world by providing the tools and great support. Partnering with ORGANIC INDIA gives a new dimension to my original mission to clean as many people as I could.

My partnership with ORGANIC INDIA is not the result of a business decision in which I calculated how I would make more money. It is the marriage of two companies that have complementary missions. CLEAN is dedicated to cleaning the human body, ORGANIC INDIA is dedicated to cleaning the planetary body. When I tell you to use herbs on the program, I will provide the generic names. I am sure there are other companies that also make quality Ayurvedic herbs. I just know that ORGANIC INDIA herbs, which are grown and prepared according to Dr. Narendra's findings, protocol, and forty years of experience, are the best, and I have seen them work. Not only that, whenever you use these herbs, you are helping turn more land into organic regenerative farming and supporting thousands of farmers and their families. In this way, you are helping to detox and heal the planet.

I mentioned above that I see humans as the red blood cells of the planetary body. Red blood cells have an essential function for life: they carry oxygen from the lungs to every cell in the body. Humans also have a function: we are energy transformers. We get energy from oxygen, food, and impressions and we transform these into our "experience." If we are experiencing peace, or love, we are fulfilling our function. We carry that state everywhere, and just as red blood cells do with oxygen, we do with love. Whoever comes in contact will benefit, and it's essential to life. This state will also align you with nature in every sense, and you will feel more and more a part of this larger being and understand viscerally that taking care of your environment is as important as taking care of your body. In fact, they are the same thing.

7

Now What?

Congratulations!

You did it. I am so proud of you. How do you feel? It is okay to bask in the joy and pride you feel after setting your mind to do something great for yourself and then accomplishing it. The best part is that by now you are an expert in what makes you feel and look good. It's not easy to do what you just did, interrupting deeply ingrained habits that make up life as you know it. Questioning anything is courageous, but the very fabric of how you behave hour by hour is heroic. By interrupting these habits, you also interrupted the inner bombardment of toxic chemicals in your diet as well as toxic chemicals in your environment, and you supported the body's detoxification processes that reduce the backlogged overload in your body. You did this by following an elimination diet, rich in the nutrients needed to detox and added the Ayurvedic dosha personalization to optimize the energetic aspect of it. You also gradually and intermittently entered the fasting state, which facilitates detox and repair. You flooded your inner environment with herbs that benefited you in many ways, including but not limited to providing nutrients, antioxidants, herbal antimicrobials, and selective prebiotics that balance every system in your body, thanks to their adaptogenic qualities. Your genes recognized the conditions you created with the CLEAN7 program and shifted from directing your neuro-endocrine-immune systems to adapt to injury and survive, into cellular activities that result in healing, repair, vibrancy, and even rejuvenation. You may have lost weight, but even more likely, you lost volume—your clothes fit better. Your skin is smoother, with a healthy color and glow. Your hair is more lustrous and smooth and less of it is falling out, or none at all. Your dandruff (if you had any before) is much improved or gone. Your sleep is deeper, your mood more even and lighter, your mind sharper. Your minor symptom—such as itchy nose, sneezing, headaches, aches and pains—and your digestive problems are much improved. You are getting along with everybody better and are feeling good. You just took an inner shower—of body and mind.

Now please, don't jump back in the mud.

Before I tell you how to apply everything you learned this week and integrate it into a lifelong health plan, I have a confession to make. I fall off the wagon all the time. I sometimes struggle with the contradiction of knowing that something is bad for me but doing it anyway. Even though I know all the tools you just used so successfully, as did thousands of others, I cannot always follow what I teach. Life sometimes gets in the way. I recently went through tough times and it threw me off track. The reason I found these tools is that I needed them, and I still do. I am grateful I have them. They allow me, during bad times, to not go too deep down the rabbit hole. It is also true that the ups and downs occur less often and are less intense as time goes by, because of and thanks to these tools. I have designed CLEAN7 as the ultimate jumpstart and re-tuning program. The results should be powerful enough to give you a sense of what is possible in terms of your health. Going forward you can extend the program and always use CLEAN7 periodically, and that is exactly the doctor's order I offer you. It will be like taking inner showers often, a lifesaver if this is the only thing you do, and it will enhance and improve anything else that you do after this. In between inner showers, the CLEAN7 program can be deconstructed and its components used individually or in combination as part of your own system to design a lifelong health plan.

Using the CLEAN7 Program

Continue

You may feel so good that you don't want to stop. I hear that all the time. In fact, I always hope to hear that, because it is a great opportunity. If seven days made you feel this way, what is possible in fourteen or twenty-one days? So much. You already have the momentum; why not continue? It will certainly solidify your results and take you to the next level. But the best part is that it will set the conditions needed for you to do the reintroduction exercise. Depending on how clean you were before you started, you need to be on CLEAN7 for at least two weeks (and ideally three, if you suspect your symptoms were food related) for the reintroduction process to be very accurate. After that, you will be able to reintroduce the foods you have been avoiding, one by one, carefully observing how your body reacts to each one. The information you gather will be more accurate and more useful than any food-allergy test available. During the CLEAN7 program you have avoided certain foods (as per the Elimination Diet and your dosha). This is a very important component to the reasons that you are feeling better. You don't know exactly which of all the foods you eliminated are the culprits that caused a negative effect (toxic trigger such as a food allergy or a food sensitivity). Over seven days your body started to reverse the negative effects of any food that is a toxic trigger to you. However, it needs one more week to balance things out so that you get to the point at which reintroducing each of the avoided foods one at a time will identify your toxic triggers, so you can plan to avoid them or decide how frequently to eat them. This is incredibly useful. Elimination (for at least two weeks) and controlled reintroduction is the best and most accurate way to determine which foods to avoid (for more detailed instructions on the correct way to complete the reintroduction phase visit www.cleanprogram.com/clean7). In my experience, after using hundreds of these lab tests with patients, I understand that these tests are at best confusing and at worse they can negatively impact people's lives. They measure immunoglobulins that match the antigens of certain foods, but that is not the only mechanism by which foods may negatively impact the body. There are also often false positives, meaning that the immunoglobulins are there but no real allergy. People may get scared to eat something that they don't really have to avoid. Besides, reactions to food depend on the health of your intestines. For example, you may react very negatively to a food if your gut flora is unhealthy, and once your gut flora normalizes, that food sensitivity may disappear. It is wise to do the elimination/reintroduction (E/R) exercise periodically. How often is difficult to say. It is not so much a matter of time, but how you are feeling. If your health turns in a bad direction, that's a time to do it. When you are back to feeling well, that is when you can do it again, so you can safely reintroduce the foods you've been avoiding while you were getting better. Over time, you learn so much about your body and how it reacts to foods that the E/R becomes more and more limited to only a few things, and you will be able to predict them correctly most of the time anyway. It is as if a personalized version of this exercise becomes embedded in your habits. Please note that even if you don't follow the protocol of liquid-solid meals for the next week, and just follow the dietary guidelines, you will benefit from the E/R exercise. If you want to go deeper, continue for two more weeks. In *CLEAN,* I provide a twenty-one-day program. In that book, I explain why twenty-one days is such an important threshold for achieving long-lasting results. There are many ways in which you can do this. You can repeat the CLEAN7 program all over again or you can add a level of difficulty each week to take things even further. Please refer to chapter 7, where you will find examples of different levels of CLEAN7 as well as the principles you need to know to tone it up or down, according to where you stand. Another option is to simply complete the next two weeks by sliding over to the original program.

I am always asked "how long is it safe to do the program continuously"? It is safer to be on the CLEAN7 protocol for life than on Standard American Diet and Schedule.

Repeat Periodically

Use the CLEAN7 program as you do a shower, periodically and as frequently as needed. If you stay clean between showers, you will need to shower less often. On average, a week of CLEAN7 every change of season is ideal. But you be the judge. Try it, play with it. You have the rest of your life to learn.

Build Your Own Level of Difficulty

Design your personalized CLEAN7 program.

1. Print a few copies of this program illustration.

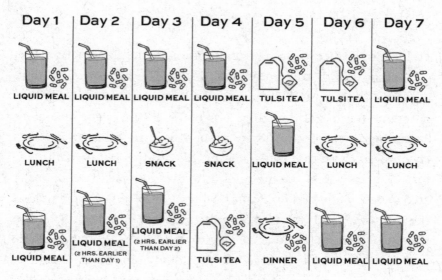

A liquid meal can be a shake, a smoothie, or a soup.

2. Cut down the lines so you end up with a few strips for each day (a few day one strips, a few day two strips, and so on, for each day).

3. Design your own program by using these strips in any combination that makes sense to you and repeating certain days. For example, you may repeat days 4 and 5 if you decide to include two twenty-four-hour fasts into your week. By looking at the week and thinking it through as you consider the principles you've learned, you can design a whole spectrum of difficulties.

Deconstructing CLEAN7

The CLEAN7 program is designed to include many principles that complement each other but can also be used individually.

CLEAN7 Diet

The CLEAN7 diet is the personalization of the Elimination Diet (ED) according to your individual dosha. The benefit of combining these two forms of dietary advice is specific to benefit a detox program. While not detoxing, it is better to use them separately. According to the dosha system alone, there are foods that one is encouraged to eat that, when combined with the ED, are contradictory. Dairy is one of the main foods to avoid in the ED but considered beneficial for certain doshas. Your CLEAN7 diet simply reflects the list of the foods to avoid according to the Elimination Diet *plus* the list of foods to avoid according to your dosha. If you decide to explore the complete Ayurvedic nutritional approach, it would be ideal to have a consultation with an Ayurvedic practitioner or visit www.cleanprogram.com/clean7 for more on ways to use this incredible system to keep you vibrantly healthy.

In the meantime, repeat the questionnaire choosing your answers according to how you feel today and find out if your starting vikriti has shifted. If not, you can continue following those guidelines. If your vikriti shifted, it may be time to go back to following your primordial dosha (prakriti) general guidelines.

The
CLEAN7
Tools

The CLEAN7 Tools

Your CLEAN7 Planner

There is no single way to organize and accomplish CLEAN7. If you're not a big planner, you may prefer to simply look at the recipes day by day. I do advise you to have all the ingredients you will need for the week at hand. (See pages 194–271 for recipes for the three doshas.) Those of you who prefer more structure will benefit from writing a plan in advance, using the following chart. You can download a copy of this planner at www.cleanprogram.com/clean7. Planning can not only save you time, it can also help you stay focused and accountable for your actions. However you decide to proceed, please read the material in this section first. It will walk you through the CLEAN7 program.

Here's what I suggest: Pick out the recipes suitable for your dosha for the week, being realistic but as adventurous as possible. Make a shopping list of the ingredients you'll need, including herbs and supplements. Even if you don't stick to the exact recipe plan, you'll be well supplied for a variety of CLEAN7 meals. Fill out the planner, jotting down as a reminder any supplements and herbs you will be using. Also indicate any optional practices you want to include, such as a massage, yoga classes, a sauna, or a colonic outside the home. Jot down reminders of things you might forget about, like taking time to write down your thoughts or meditate. Post your chart on the fridge or somewhere you will see it daily.

YOUR CLEAN7 PLANNER

DAY 1

Shake: _____

_____

Lunch: _____

_____

Shake: _____

_____

Herbs: _____

_____

Appointments: _____

_____

Checklist:

❏ Filtered Water   ❏ Skin Brushing

❏ Sleep/Rest   ❏ Hot/Cold Plunge

❏ 5-Minute Meditation   ❏ Enema/Colonic

❏ Mindful Breathing   ❏ Massage/Acupuncture

❏ Journaling   ❏ Sauna/Steam

❏ Exercise/Movement

Reminders: _____

_____

DAY 2

Shake: _____

_____

Lunch: _____

_____

Shake: _____

_____

Herbs: _____

_____

Appointments: _____

_____

Checklist:

❑ Filtered Water   ❑ Skin Brushing

❑ Sleep/Rest   ❑ Hot/Cold Plunge

❑ 5-Minute Meditation   ❑ Enema/Colonic

❑ Mindful Breathing   ❑ Massage/Acupuncture

❑ Journaling   ❑ Sauna/Steam

❑ Exercise/Movement

Reminders: _____

_____

DAY 3

Shake: _____
_____

Snack: _____
_____

Shake: _____
_____

Herbs: _____
_____

Appointments: _____
_____

Checklist:

❏ Filtered Water   ❏ Skin Brushing

❏ Sleep/Rest   ❏ Hot/Cold Plunge

❏ 5-Minute Meditation   ❏ Enema/Colonic

❏ Mindful Breathing   ❏ Massage/Acupuncture

❏ Journaling   ❏ Sauna/Steam

❏ Exercise/Movement

Reminders: _____
_____

DAY 4

Shake: _____
_____

Snack: _____

_____

Tulsi tea: _____

_____

Herbs: _____

_____

Appointments: _____

_____

Checklist:

❑ Filtered Water   ❑ Skin Brushing

❑ Sleep/Rest   ❑ Hot/Cold Plunge

❑ 5-Minute Meditation   ❑ Enema/Colonic

❑ Mindful Breathing   ❑ Massage/Acupuncture

❑ Journaling   ❑ Sauna/Steam

❑ Exercise/Movement

Reminders: _____

_____

DAY 5

Tulsi tea: _____
_____

Shake: _____
_____

Dinner: _____
_____

Herbs: _____
_____

Appointments: _____
_____

Checklist:

❑ Filtered Water   ❑ Skin Brushing

❑ Sleep/Rest   ❑ Hot/Cold Plunge

❑ 5-Minute Meditation   ❑ Enema/Colonic

❑ Mindful Breathing   ❑ Massage/Acupuncture

❑ Journaling   ❑ Sauna/Steam

❑ Exercise/Movement

Reminders: _____
_____

DAY 6

Tulsi tea: _____

_____

Lunch: _____

_____

Shake: _____

_____

Herbs: _____

_____

Appointments: _____

_____

Checklist:

❑ Filtered Water

❑ Sleep/Rest

❑ 5-Minute Meditation

❑ Mindful Breathing

❑ Journaling

❑ Exercise/Movement

❑ Skin Brushing

❑ Hot/Cold Plunge

❑ Enema/Colonic

❑ Massage/Acupuncture

❑ Sauna/Steam

Reminders: _____

_____

DAY 7

Shake: _____

_____

Lunch: _____

_____

Shake: _____

_____

Herbs: _____

_____

Appointments: _____

_____

Checklist:

- ❏ Filtered Water
- ❏ Sleep/Rest
- ❏ 5-Minute Meditation
- ❏ Mindful Breathing
- ❏ Journaling
- ❏ Exercise/Movement

- ❏ Skin Brushing
- ❏ Hot/Cold Plunge
- ❏ Enema/Colonic
- ❏ Massage/Acupuncture
- ❏ Sauna/Steam

Reminders: _____

_____

The CLEAN7 diet, or more specifically each of three diets, is composed of the acceptable foods on the Elimination Diet plus the foods recommended for each dosha. Following are the foods to avoid and enjoy for each dosha. Starting on page 164 you will find lists of recommended foods and foods to avoid that integrate the Elimination Diet with each of the three doshas. But first you need to find your dosha by answering the questions on the following questionnaire.

THE CLEAN DIET: THE COMPLETE LIST

Foods to Enjoy

Fruits & Vegetables	Unsweetened fresh or frozen whole fruits, sea vegetables (seaweeds), avocados, olives, tubers (sweet potatoes, yams), and raw, steamed, sauteed, juiced, or roasted vegetables
Dairy Substitutes	Hemp and nut milks (such as almond, hazelnut, walnut, etc.), coconut milk, coconut oil/butter
Starch & Non-Gluten Grains	Brown, red, black and wild rice, millet, amaranth, teff, tapioca (including cassava), buckwheat, quinoa
Animal Protein	Fresh or water-packed cold-water fish (trout, salmon, halibut, tuna, mackerel, sardines, pike, kippers), wild game (rabbit, pheasant, bison, venison, elk, etc.), lamb, duck, organic chicken, turkey, collagen, bone broth
Vegetable Protein	Split peas, lentils, legumes, bee pollen, spirulina, blue-green algae
Nuts & Seeds	Hemp, chia, flax, sesame, pumpkin, and sunflower seeds, hazelnuts, pecans, almonds, walnuts, cashews, macadamia, pistachios, Brazil, nut and seed butters, such as almond or tahini
Oils	Cold-pressed olive, coconut, flax, safflower, sesame, almond, sunflower, walnut, pumpkin, avocado
Drinks	Filtered water, green, white or herbal tea, unflavored seltzer or mineral water, yerba maté, coconut water, green juice
Sweeteners	Stevia, monkfruit extract, coconut sugar/nectar, xylitol, whole/fresh fruit
Condiments	Vinegar, all spices, all herbs, Himalayan or sea salt, black pepper, carob, raw or dark chocolate (dairy and sugar free), stone-ground mustard, miso, coconut liquid aminos, wheat-free tamari and nama shoyu, unsweetened whole fruit jam

In moderation:
powdered cayenne, kombucha, dried fruit, and snacking.

Foods to Avoid

Oranges, grapefruit, bananas, strawberries, grapes/raisins, corn, creamed vegetables, nightshades (goji berries, tomatoes, peppers, eggplant, regular potatoes)

Dairy and eggs, including milk, cheese, cottage cheese, cream, yogurt, butter, ice cream, nondairy creamers, ghee, soy milk

White rice, wheat, corn, barley, spelt, kamut, rye, triticale, oats (even gluten-free)

Pork (bacon), beef, veal, sausage, cold cuts, canned meats, frankfurters (hot dogs), shellfish, any raw meats, raw fish, sushi, warm-water fish

Soybean products (tofu, soy sauce, soybean oil in processed foods)

Peanuts and peanut butter

Butter, margarine, shortening, processed oils, canola oil, salad dressings, mayonnaise, spreads

Alcohol, coffee (including decaf), non-approved caffeinated beverages, soft drinks, fruit juice (unless fresh pressed)

Refined sugar, white/brown sugars, maple syrup, high-fructose corn syrup, evaporated cane juice, Splenda®, Equal®, Sweet'N Low®, juice concentrate, agave nectar, brown rice syrup, honey

Regular chocolate (with dairy and sugar), ketchup, hot sauce, relish, chutney, traditional soy sauce, barbecue sauce, teriyaki sauce, breath mints, chewing gum

It's important to check labels and ingredients of foods.
Use grass-fed, organic, or free-range when possible.

FIND YOUR DOSHA QUESTIONNAIRE

To determine your constitution it is best to fill out the chart twice. First, base your choices on what is most consistent over a long period of your life (your prakriti), then fill it out a second time responding to how you have been feeling more recently (your vikriti). Sometimes it helps to have a friend ask you the questions and fill in the chart for you, as they may have insight (and impartiality) to offer. After finishing the chart each time, add up the number of marks under vata, pitta, and kapha.

OBSERVATIONS	V	P	K	VATA
Body size	❑	❑	❑	Slim
Body weight	❑	❑	❑	Low
Chin	❑	❑	❑	Thin, angular
Cheeks	❑	❑	❑	Wrinkled, sunken
Eyes	❑	❑	❑	Small, sunken, dry, active, black, brown, nervous Uneven shape, deviated
Nose	❑	❑	❑	Uneven shape, deviated septum
Lips	❑	❑	❑	Dry, cracked, black/brown tinge
Teeth	❑	❑	❑	Stick out, big, roomy, thin gums
Skin	❑	❑	❑	Thin, dry, cold, rough, dark
Hair	❑	❑	❑	Dry brown, black, knotted, brittle, scarce
Nails	❑	❑	❑	Dry, rough, brittle, break easily
Neck	❑	❑	❑	Thin, tall
Chest	❑	❑	❑	Flat, sunken
Belly	❑	❑	❑	Thin, flat, sunken
Belly-button	❑	❑	❑	Small, irregular, herniated
Hips	❑	❑	❑	Slender, thin
Joints	❑	❑	❑	Cold, cracking
Appetite	❑	❑	❑	Irregular, scanty
Digestion	❑	❑	❑	Irregular, forms gas
Taste	❑	❑	❑	Sweet, sour, salty
Thirst	❑	❑	❑	Changeable
Elimination	❑	❑	❑	Constipation
Physical Activity	❑	❑	❑	Hyperactive
Mental Activity	❑	❑	❑	Hyperactive
Emotions	❑	❑	❑	Anxiety, fear, uncertainty
Faith	❑	❑	❑	Variable
Intellect	❑	❑	❑	Quick but faulty response
Recollection	❑	❑	❑	Recent good, remote poor
Dreams	❑	❑	❑	Quick, active, many, fearful
Sleep	❑	❑	❑	Scanty, broken up, sleeplessness
Speech	❑	❑	❑	Rapid, unclear
Financial	❑	❑	❑	Poor, spends on trifles
TOTAL				

This will help you discover your own ratio of doshas in your prakriti and vikriti. Most people will have one dosha predominant, a few will have two doshas approximately equal, and even fewer will have all three doshas in equal proportion. For instance, if your vikriti shows more pitta than your prakriti, you will want to follow a pitta-soothing regimen to try and bring your vikriti back into balance with your prakriti. If your prakriti and vikriti seem about the same, then you would choose the regimen of your strongest dosha.

PITTA	KAPHA
Medium	Large
Medium	Overweight
Tapering	Rounded, double
Smooth flat	Rounded, plump
Sharp, bright, gray, green, yellow/red, sensitive to light	Big, beautiful, blue, calm, loving
Long pointed, red nose tip	Short rounded, button nose
Red, inflamed, yellowish	Smooth, oily, pale, whitish
Medium, soft, tender gums	Healthy, white, strong gums
Smooth, oily, warm, rosy	Thick, oily, cool, white, pale
Straight, oily, blond, gray, red, bald	Thick, curly, oily, wavy, luxuriant
Sharp, flexible, pink, lustrous	Thick, oily, smooth, polished
Medium	Big, folded
Moderate	Expanded, round
Moderate	Big, pot-bellied
Oval, superficial	Big, deep, round, stretched
Moderate	Heavy, big
Moderate	Large, lubricated
Strong, unbearable	Slow but steady
Quick, causes burning	Prolonged, forms mucous
Sweet, bitter, astringent	Bitter, pungent, astringent
Surplus	Sparse
Loose	Thick, oily, sluggish
Moderate	Slow
Moderate	Dull, slow
Anger, hate, jealousy	Calm, greedy, attachment
Extremist	Consistent
Accurate response	Slow, exact
Distinct	Slow and sustained
Fiery, war, violence	Lakes, snow, romantic
Little but sound	Deep, prolonged
Sharp, penetrating	Slow, monotonous
Spends money on luxuries	Rich, good money preserver

© 1994, 2019 excerpt from *Ayurvedic Cooking for Self-Healing* by Usha and Dr. Lad
The Ayurvedic Institute • 11311 Menaul Blvd NE •
Albuquerque, NM 87112-0008 • (505) 291-9698 • www.ayurveda.com

FOOD LISTS FOR THE THREE DOSHAS

The following lists of foods for each of the three doshas clarify which foods you should be eating, which you should avoid, and which should be consumed in moderation. The recipes that start on page 194, organized by dosha, comply with these guidelines. The lists should also guide you in making your own dosha-specific recipes and in making grocery shopping list for your week on CLEAN7. The lists of foods to avoid and foods to enjoy

CHART 1:
VATA DOSHA FOODS TO ENJOY
AND FOODS TO AVOID

In general, eat warm, moist, cooked meals, prepared by steaming,

Foods to Enjoy

Most sweet fruits such as apples (cooked), apricots, cherries, lemons, limes, mangos, papayas, peaches, and papaya; also avocado and rhubarb

Most vegetables except listed on page 155; in general, most vegetables should be cooked; cooked cabbage, cauliflower, onions, peas, and radishes; raw daikon radish, lettuce, spinach, parsley, and most other leafy greens should be consumed in moderation, as well as chili peppers and coriander leaves

Quinoa, basmati and other types of rice, amaranth*

Mung beans, mung dal

Most dairy (see page 154 for more detail)

Free-range chicken (dark meat) and turkey (dark meat); beef, bison, duck, eggs

Freshwater and ocean fish, including shrimp

All nuts and pumpkin, sunflower, and most other seeds

are based upon (and used with permission) a more complete list compiled by The Ayurvedic Institute based in Santa Fe, New Mexico (www.ayurveda .com). Understand that because Ayurveda is such an ancient program, there is a fair amount of variation from one source to another. If you purchase an Ayurvedic cookbook or visit another website, you might find somewhat different guidelines for each dosha.

---

sautéing, and roasting. Cooked vegetables are best. Minimize intake of all raw veggies as well as both cooked and raw cabbage and sprouts. Cook with olive oil—try to have a tablespoon of extra-virgin olive oil each day—sesame and most other oils. All spices are fine, but use black pepper, cayenne, and fenugreek in moderation.

Foods to Avoid

Raisins, dried dates, and most other dried fruits and raw apples; also cranberries, pears, persimmons, pomegranate, and watermelon

Raw vegetables such as onion, cabbage, radish, peas, and cauliflower

Buckwheat

Kidney beans, adzuki beans, brown lentils, and most other legumes

Turkey (white meat), lamb, pork, rabbit, venison

Chocolate, horseradish

Psyllium seeds

Foods with an asterisk (*) should be eaten only in moderation.

CHART 2:
PITTA DOSHA FOODS TO ENJOY AND FOODS TO AVOID

Foods to Enjoy

Avocados and sweet fruits such as cherries, melons, coconut, pomegranate, mango, sweet berries, and fully ripened pineapple and plums; also limes*

Sweet and bitter vegetables such as asparagus, cucumber, sweet potato, lettuce and other leafy greens, pumpkin, broccoli, cauliflower, celery, okra, green beans, and zucchini; also watercress* and raw carrots*

Amaranth; quinoa; and basmati, white, and wild rice

All legumes except tur dal and urad dal

Freshwater fish, shrimp*

White-meat chicken and turkey, buffalo, venison, rabbit, egg whites

Soaked almonds, coconut

Sunflower, ghee, canola, coconut, olive oil, soy, flaxseed, primrose, walnut, almond oils

Flaxseeds, psyllium, pumpkin*, and sunflower seeds

In general, avoid very spicy, salty, and oily foods and use spices such as fenugreek, cardamom, and coriander. Use black pepper and chili peppers in moderation. It is best to cook with olive or sunflower seed oils. You can also use walnut oil to dress vegetables.

Foods to Avoid

Sour fruits such as sour apples or apricots, cranberries, kiwi, green mangos, lime, rhubarb, and tamarind

Pungent vegetables such as hot peppers, beets, onions, garlic, radishes, and raw spinach

Buckwheat and millet

Dark-meat chicken and turkey, lamb, ocean fish

Chili peppers, chocolate, horseradish, lemon, vinegar, pickles, excessively salty or hot foods and condiments

Almonds (with skin), black walnuts, Brazil nuts, cashews, filberts, hazelnuts, macadamias

Pecans, pine nuts, pistachios, and walnuts

Chia and sesame seeds, tahini

Foods with an asterisk (*) should be eaten only in moderation.

CHART 3:
KAPHA DOSHA FOODS TO ENJOY
AND FOODS TO AVOID

Foods to Enjoy

Most astringent fruit such as apples, apricots, berries, cherries, cranberries, dry figs, grapes*, lemons*, limes*, peaches*, pears, persimmon, pomegranate, and raisins

Most pungent and bitter vegetables such as artichokes, asparagus, beets and their greens, broccoli, Brussels sprouts, cabbage, carrots, cauliflower, celery, daikon, fennel, garlic, green beans, green chilies, horseradish, Jerusalem artichokes, kale, kohlrabi, leafy greens, mustard greens, okra, onions, parsley, peas, peppers (sweet and hot), radishes, spaghetti squash*, spinach, winter squash, turnips and their greens, and watercress

Amaranth, barley, buckwheat, cold cereal, corn, couscous, millet, oats, quinoa, rye, basmati and wild rice, wheat, spelt*

Almost all legumes, including mung beans*, mung dal*, soy, hot tofu*

Buttermilk*, cottage cheese from skim goat milk, ghee*, goat cheese (unsalted and unaged), goat milk, skim goat milk yogurt (diluted)

Corn, canola, sunflower, and almond oils; ghee

White-meat chicken and turkey, rabbit, venison, freshwater fish, shrimp, eggs

Chia, flax, pumpkin*, and sunflower seeds; popcorn (without butter and salt)

In general, consume warm, lightly cooked food, preferably baked, broiled, grilled, or sautéed, and lots of raw vegetables and fruit. Select hot food over cold whenever possible. Avoid heavy meals and have your main meal in the middle of the day. Reduce your intake of all nuts and seeds. Cook only with sunflower seed oil. Fruit should generally be astringent rather than sweet or sour. Preferred spices are fenugreek, ginger, and black pepper.

Foods to Avoid

Avocado, bananas, coconut, dates, fresh figs, grapefruit, kiwi, mangos (okay rarely), melons, oranges, papaya, pineapple, plums, rhubarb, tamarind, and watermelon

Sweet and juicy veggies such as cucumber, olives, parsnips, sweet potatoes, pumpkin, taro root, zucchini and other summer squash

Brown and white rice, rice cakes wheat, bread, oats, pasta (okay rarely)

Kidney beans, urad dal, soy beans and soy products, miso, cold tofu

Dark-meat chicken or turkey, duck; beef, bison, lamb, pork

All wild-caught fish, salmon, sardines, tuna, and other seafood

Butter, cheese, cow's milk, ice cream, sour cream, yogurt

Chocolate, salt, sugar, tamari, vinegar

All nuts and sesame seeds, tahini

Foods with an asterisk (*) should be eaten only in moderation.

CHART 4:
COMBINED ELIMINATION DIET AND VATA DOSHA FOODS TO ENJOY AND FOODS TO AVOID

Foods to Enjoy

Vegetables	In general, most vegetables should be cooked (steamed, sautéed, or roasted), including asparagus, beets, cabbage*, carrots, cauliflower*, cilantro, cucumber, daikon radish*, fennel, garlic, green beans, Jerusalem artichoke*, leeks, lettuce, mustard greens*, okra, black olives, onions*, parsley*, parsnips, peas, sweet potatoes and yams, pumpkin, radishes (cooked)*, rutabaga, spaghetti squash*, spinach*, sprouts*, summer squash, taro root, turnip greens*, watercress, and zucchini; raw leafy greens such as lettuce*, watercress, spinach*, and parsley
Fruits	In general, most sweet fruit, including cooked apples, apricots, avocado, most berries but not strawberries, sweet cherries, coconut, fresh dates, fresh figs, kiwi, lemons, limes, mangos, melons, papaya, peaches, pineapple, plums, soaked prunes*, rhubarb, and tamarind; fresh-squeezed juice from acceptable fruits
Dairy Substitutes	Hemp, rice, and nut "milk" beverages, such as almond, coconut, hazelnut, walnut, and cashew; unsweetened canned coconut milk
Grains	Brown, red, black, basmati, and wild rice amaranth*, teff, and quinoa
Animal Protein	Fresh or water-packed cold-water fish such as halibut, herring, mackerel, pike, sardines, salmon, trout, and tuna; duck, white-* and dark-meat chicken, and dark-meat turkey
Vegetable Protein	Chickpeas (garbanzo beans)*, mung beans, mung dal, tur dal, urad dal

All foods listed are suitable for both the Elimination Diet and Vata dosha.

Nuts & Seeds	Black walnuts*, Brazil nuts*, cashews*, coconut*, filberts*, hazelnuts*, macadamia nuts*, pecans*, pine nuts*, pistachios*, and walnuts*; chia, hemp, flax, pumpkin, sesame, and sunflower seeds; almond butter and tahini
Oils	Cold-pressed extra-virgin olive oil (to dress vegetables); almond, avocado, coconut, sesame, almond, walnut, and pumpkin oils
Beverages	Filtered, distilled, or mineral water; decaffeinated herbal teas and tulsi, yerba maté, green, white, and red teas; almond milk, coconut milk, rice milk; aloe vera juice*, apple cider, fresh-squeezed juice (not from concentrate) such as apricot, some berries (except for strawberry), carrot*, mango, papaya, and pineapple juice (but no cranberry, cherry, grape, grapefruit, orange, or other citrus juices); soy-free miso broth*
Sweeteners	Stevia
Condiments	Vinegar, wheat-free tamari, soy-free miso, and coconut liquid aminos, lemons and limes; all spices (except cayenne, paprika, and chili powder or chili flakes), including cinnamon, cumin, ginger, Himalayan pink salt and sea salt, and black pepper*; all herbs, including dill, oregano, parsley, rosemary, tarragon, thyme, and turmeric; garlic, cooked onions*, and scallions; seaweed: kelp, dulse, gomasio, hijiki, and kombu; unsweetened stone-ground mustard, agar-agar (as a thickening agent), baking soda

Foods with an asterisk (*) should be eaten only in moderation.

Foods to Avoid

Vegetables	In general, frozen, raw, or dried vegetables; sweet corn, creamed vegetables, frozen vegetables in sauces, and fried vegetables; nightshade family vegetables: tomatoes, goji berries, sweet and hot peppers, eggplant, okra, tomatillos, and "regular" white (not sweet) potatoes; artichoke, beet greens*, bitter melon, broccoli, Brussels sprouts, burdock root, raw cabbage, raw cauliflower, celery, dandelion greens, kale, kohlrabi, mushrooms, green olives, raw onions, raw peas, prickly pear, raw radish, winter squash, turnips
Fruits	Raw apples, bananas, cherries, cranberries, grapefruit, grapes, oranges, orange juice (and other citrus juice), pears, persimmons, pomegranates, strawberries, and watermelon; canned fruits in syrup and sweetened frozen fruits; dried dates, dried figs, raisins, and prunes
Dairy & Eggs	All cow, goat, and sheep dairy, including milk, cream, butter, cheese, yogurt, whey, ghee, and ice cream; powdered cow's milk and powdered goat's milk; eggs and packaged egg whites; butter substitutes (margarine) and mayonnaise
Grains	White rice, brown rice cakes*; wheat, bread made with yeast, kamut, spelt, triticale, wheat bran, oat bran, and pasta; barley, buckwheat, corn, oats, rye, couscous, and polenta; crackers, dry breakfast cereals, granola, muesli, millet, sago, tapioca
Animal Protein	Any raw meat; any cooked beef, lamb, pork (including bacon), rabbit, veal, venison; also sausages, cold cuts, canned meats, and frankfurters (hot dogs), white-meat turkey; all shellfish, raw or cooked, including shrimp, lobster, oysters, and clams; any raw fish (sushi), farm-raised fish, and warm-water fish such as tilapia

All foods listed are excluded from either or both the Elimination Diet and Vata dosha.

Vegetable Protein	Soy beans, soy sauce, soy flour, soy powder, soy cheese, soy sausages, processed foods that contain soy or soybean oil, miso (except soy-free), tempeh, seitan, tofu, soy milk, soy yogurt, and textured vegetable protein (TVP); adzuki beans, black beans, black-eyed peas, chickpeas (garbanzo beans)*, kidney beans, brown lentils, lima beans, navy beans, dried peas, split peas, pinto beans, and white beans
Nuts & Seeds	Peanuts and peanut butter, psyllium*
Oils	Flaxseed, shortening, processed oils such as soy, canola, corn, and safflower; most store-bought salad dressings, and mayonnaise
Beverages	All hard alcohol, wine, and beer; all juices made from concentrates, apple juice, cranberry juice, orange juice, grapefruit juice, pear juice, pomegranate juice, prune juice*, tomato juice, V8 juice, and lemonade; coffee, other caffeinated beverages and black tea; carbonated drinks, soft drinks, and flavored bottled water; chocolate milk and hot cocoa; cold dairy and other cold drinks and iced tea, soy milk
Sweeteners	White sugar, refined brown sugar, honey, maple syrup, high-fructose corn syrup, agave nectar, evaporated cane juice, brown rice syrup, and juice concentrates, yacon, xylitol, Splenda, Equal, and Sweet'N Low
Condiments	All chocolate, including dark chocolate and sugar-free chocolate; horseradish, ketchup, relish, sweet or sour chutney, jams and jellies made with sugar, barbecue sauce, soy sauce, and teriyaki sauce; breath mints and chewing gum, including sugarless gum

Foods with an asterisk (*) should be eaten only rarely.

CHART 5:
COMBINED ELIMINATION DIET AND PITTA DOSHA FOODS TO ENJOY AND FOODS TO AVOID

Foods to Enjoy

Vegetables	Raw, steamed, sautéed, juiced, or roasted vegetables, including sweet and bitter vegetables such as artichokes, asparagus, cooked beets, bitter melon, broccoli, Brussels sprouts, cabbage, cooked carrots, raw carrots*, cauliflower, celery, cilantro, cucumber, dandelion greens, fennel, green beans, Jerusalem artichoke, kale, leafy greens, cooked leeks, lettuce, mushrooms, black olives, raw onions*, cooked onions, parsley, parsnips, peas, sweet potatoes, prickly pear, pumpkin, raw radishes*, cooked radishes, rutabaga, spaghetti squash, winter and summer squash, mild sprouts, spicy sprouts, taro root, watercress*, and zucchini
Fruits	Most unsweetened fresh fruit, including sweet apples, sweet apricots, avocado, all berries (except strawberries), sweet cherries, coconut, dates, figs, limes*, melons, papaya*, pears, ripe pineapple, sweet plums, pomegranate,* prunes, and watermelon; fresh-squeezed juice; dried fruit in moderation
Dairy Substitutes	Hemp, rice, and nut "milk" beverages, such as almond and coconut; unsweetened canned coconut milk; coconut oil, coconut butter
Grains	Basmati rice, brown rice*, wild rice, and brown rice cakes*, amaranth, quinoa, tapioca, and teff
Animal Protein	Freshwater and water-packed cold-water fish such as trout and salmon; rabbit, pheasant, venison, elk, and other wild game; white-meat chicken and white-meat turkey

All foods listed are suitable for both the Elimination Diet and Pitta dosha.

Vegetable Protein	Adzuki beans, black beans, black-eyed peas, chickpeas (garbanzos), kidney beans, brown and red lentils, lima beans, mung beans, mung dal, navy beans, dried peas, pinto beans, split peas, and white beans
Nuts & Seeds	Almonds (blanched) and coconut; flaxseeds, hemp seeds, psyllium*, pumpkin seeds, and sunflower seeds
Oils	Almond, flaxseed, extra-virgin olive*, avocado*, coconut, and walnut oils
Beverages	Filtered, distilled, or mineral water; decaffeinated herbal teas and tulsi, yerba maté, green white, and red teas; almond milk; fresh-squeezed aloe vera juice; apple, apricot, sweet berry, cherry, mango, pear, pineapple, pomegranate*, and prune juice*; miso broth (soy-free)
Sweeteners	Stevia
Condiments	Vinegar; all spices (except paprika, chili powder, chili flakes, and cayenne), including cinnamon, cumin, ginger, sea salt*, and black pepper*; all herbs, including cilantro, dill, oregano, parsley, rosemary, tarragon, thyme, and turmeric; carob, seaweed*, dulse*, hijiki*, and kombu*, unsweetened stone-ground mustard, soy-free miso, coconut liquid aminos, and wheat-free tamari sauce*; lime*, agar-agar (as a thickening agent), baking soda

Foods with an asterisk (*) should be eaten only in moderation.

Foods to Avoid

Vegetables	Sweet corn, creamed vegetables, frozen vegetables in sauces, fried vegetables; nightshade family vegetables: tomatoes, tomatillos, okra, goji berries, sweet and hot peppers, eggplant, and "regular" (not sweet) potatoes; pungent vegetables such as beet greens, raw beets; burdock root, daikon radish, garlic, horseradish, raw leeks, mustard greens, green olives, raw onions, prickly pear, raw radishes, raw spinach, and turnips and turnip greens
Fruits	Sour fruits such as sour apples, sour apricots, sour berries, sour cherries, cranberries, kiwi, green mangos*, lemons, sour pineapple, sour plums, rhubarb, and tamarind; bananas, grapefruit, grapes, oranges and other citrus, strawberries, peaches, persimmons, and raisins; canned fruits in syrup and sweetened frozen fruits
Dairy & Eggs	All cow, goat, and sheep dairy, including all cheese, butter, ghee, sour cream, whey, yogurt, and ice cream; eggs and packaged egg whites; butter substitutes (margarine) and mayonnaise
Grains	Brown rice*, buckwheat, wheat, corn, barley, spelt, kamut, millet, oats, polenta, rye, triticale, and oat; bread made with yeast
Animal Protein	Any raw meat and any pork (including bacon), beef, bison, sausages, cold cuts, canned meats, frankfurters (hot), dark-meat chicken, dark-meat turkey, duck; shellfish, raw or cooked, including shrimp, lobster, oysters, and clams; any raw fish (sushi), farm-raised fish, ocean fish/seafood such as tuna, sardines, and salmon

All foods listed are excluded from either or both the Elimination Diet and Pitta dosha.

Vegetable Protein	All soybean products: miso, soy sauce, soy or soybean oil in processed foods, tempeh, tofu, soy milk, soy sausages, soy yogurt, textured vegetable protein (TVP), tur dal, and urad dal
Nuts & Seeds	Almonds with skin, black walnuts, Brazil nuts, cashews, filberts, hazelnuts, macadamia nuts, peanuts and peanut butter, pecans, pine nuts, pistachios, and walnuts; chia seeds, sesame seeds, tahini
Oils	Almond, apricot, corn, safflower, sesame, shortening, all processed oils, canola oil, most salad dressings, mayonnaise, and margarine spreads
Beverages	All hard alcohol, wine, and beer; apple cider; carrot juice, sour cherry juice, cranberry juice, grapefruit juice, lemonade, papaya juice, pineapple juice, tomato juice, V8 juice, and any sour juice; any fruit juice unless fresh pressed; coffee or other caffeinated beverages and black stead; icy cold drinks and iced tea; carbonated beverages, sodas, soft drinks, and flavored bottled water; chocolate milk and hot cocoa
Sweeteners	White sugar, refined brown sugar, including jaggery (a form of brown sugar); honey, maple syrup, high-fructose corn syrup, agave nectar, evaporated cane juice, brown rice syrup, and juice concentrates; coconut nectar, yacón, xylitol, Splenda, Equal, and Sweet'N Low
Condiments	Chili pepper, barbecue sauce, all chocolate (including sugar free), mango chutney and any chutney, horseradish, ketchup, relish, most jams and jellies (made with sugar), mustard, lemon, lime pickle, mango pickle, mayonnaise, all pickles, excessive salt, kelp, and gomasio, and teriyaki sauce; breath mints and chewing gum (including sugarless gum)

Foods with an asterisk (*) should be eaten only rarely.

CHART 6:
COMBINED ELIMINATION DIET AND KAPHA DOSHA FOODS TO ENJOY AND FOODS TO AVOID

Foods to Enjoy

Vegetables	Raw, steamed, sautéed, juiced, or roasted vegetables; in general, most pungent and bitter vegetables: artichokes, asparagus, beets, beet greens, bitter melon, broccoli, Brussels sprouts, burdock root, cabbage, carrots, cauliflower, celery, cilantro, daikon radish, dandelion greens, fennel, garlic, green beans, horseradish, Jerusalem artichoke, kale, leafy greens, leeks, lettuce, mushrooms, mustard greens, onions, parsley, peas, prickly pear, radishes, rutabaga, spaghetti squash*, spinach, winter squash, sprouts, turnip greens, turnips, and watercress
Fruits	Unsweetened fresh fruit, fresh-squeezed juice, and frozen whole fruit without added sugar; dried fruit* (but no raisins); in general, astringent fruits such as apples, apricots, all berries except strawberries, cherries, cranberries, dried figs*, lemons*, limes*, peaches*, pears, papaya, persimmons, pomegranates, plums, and prunes*
Dairy Substitutes	Flaxseed "milk" beverage
Grains	Basmati rice and wild rice*; amaranth*, buckwheat, millet, quinoa*, and tapioca
Animal Protein	Rabbit and venison; white-meat chicken and white-meat turkey; wild-caught fish such as trout, salmon, and pike

All foods listed are suitable for both the Elimination Diet and Pitta dosha.

Vegetable Protein	Adzuki beans, black beans, black-eyed peas, chickpeas (garbanzo beans), brown and red lentils, lima beans, mung beans*, mung dal*, navy beans, dried peas, pinto beans, split peas, tur dal, and white beans
Nuts & Seeds	Chia seeds, flaxseeds*, pumpkin seeds, and sunflower seeds*
Oils	Almond and sunflower oils
Beverages	Filtered, distilled, or mineral water; decaffeinated herbal teas and tulsi, yerba maté, and green, white, and red teas; flaxseed milk; fresh-squeezed juices only: aloe vera juice; apple juice*, apple cider, apricot juice, berry juice (but not strawberry juice), carob juice, carrot juice, cherry juice, cranberry juice, mango juice, pear juice, pineapple juice*, pomegranate juice, and prune juice*
Sweeteners	Stevia
Condiments	All spices (except salt*, paprika, chili pepper, chili flakes), including cinnamon, cumin, coriander, ginger, and black pepper; all herbs, including cilantro, dill, oregano, parsley, rosemary, tarragon, thyme, and turmeric; seaweed*, dulse*, and hijiki*, unsweetened stone-ground mustard without vinegar, soy-free miso, wheat-free tamari sauce, and coconut liquid aminos*; horseradish, scallions*, lemon*, and lime*, agar-agar (as a thickening agent), baking soda

Foods with an asterisk (*) should be eaten only in moderation.

Foods to Avoid

Vegetables	Nightshade family vegetables: tomatoes, tomatillos, goji berries, okra, sweet and hot peppers, eggplant, and "regular" white potatoes; creamed vegetables, frozen vegetable in sauces, and fried vegetables; in general, sweet or juicy vegetables: cucumbers, black and green olives, parsnips*, sweet potatoes, corn, pumpkin, summer squash, taro root, and zucchini
Fruits	In general, sweet and sour fruit: avocado, bananas, coconut, cherries, dates, fresh figs, grapefruit, grapes, kiwi, mangos,* melons, oranges, papaya, pineapple, plums, raisins, rhubarb, strawberries, tamarind, and watermelon; canned fruits in syrup and sweetened frozen fruits
Dairy & Eggs	All cow, goat, and sheep dairy, including milk, cream, butter, ghee, cheese, whey, yogurt, and ice cream; eggs and packaged egg whites; butter substitutes (margarine) and mayonnaise
Grains	Brown rice, white rice (except basmati), wheat, corn, barley, spelt, kamut, rye, triticale, oats, pancakes, pasta, rye, bread made with yeast
Animal Protein	Dark-meat chicken, dark-meat turkey, and duck; any raw meat; pork (including bacon), beef, bison, lamb, and veal, sausages, cold cuts, canned meats, and frankfurters (hot dogs); shellfish, raw or cooked, including shrimp, lobster, oysters, and clams; any raw fish (sushi) or farm-raised fish; ocean fish such as tuna and sardines; also salmon

All foods listed are excluded from either or both the Elimination Diet and Pitta dosha.

Vegetable Protein	Soybean products: miso (except soy-free), soy sauce, soybean oil in processed foods, tempeh, tofu, soy cheese, soy flour, soy powder, soy sausages, soy yogurt, textured vegetable protein (TVP); urad dal and kidney beans
Nuts & Seeds	Almonds (blanched)*, black walnuts, Brazil nuts, coconut, cashews, filberts, hazelnuts, macadamia nuts, peanuts and peanut butter, pecans, pine nuts, pistachios, and walnuts, psyllium*, sesame seeds, and tahini
Oils	Avocado, coconut, apricot, olive, safflower, sesame, soy, and walnut oils; shortening; all processed oils such as canola oil, corn oil, vegetable oil; most store-bought salad dressings, mayonnaise, margarine spreads, and ghee
Beverages	Hard alcohol, beer, and wine; almond milk, rice milk, and soy milk; coffee or other caffeinated beverages*; icy-cold drinks, iced tea, and any dairy drinks; carbonated beverages, sodas, soft drinks, and flavored bottled water; grapefruit juice, lemonade, orange juice, papaya juice, tomato juice, V8 juice, and other sour juices; any fruit juice made from concentrate, chocolate milk and hot cocoa; miso broth (unless soy-free)
Sweeteners	White sugar, barley malt, evaporated cane juice, fructose, refined brown sugar, including jaggery (a form of brown sugar), honey, maple syrup, molasses, high-fructose corn syrup, agave nectar, brown rice syrup, and juice concentrates, coconut nectar, yacon, xylitol, Splenda, Equal, and Sweet'N Low
Condiments	Carob, all chocolate, cocoa nibs, all chutney, kelp and gomasio, ketchup, relish, jams and jellies made with sugar, lime, lime pickle, other pickles, mango pickle, mayonnaise, salt, soy sauce, tamari, teriyaki sauce, and vinegar; breath mints and chewing gum (including sugarless gum)

Foods with an asterisk (*) should be eaten only rarely.

Other Ways to Follow Through after Doing CLEAN7

A Shake a Day

A great way to give your body a more natural digestion-absorption-detoxification experience is to replace one meal a day with a shake. As you now know, digesting food all day long is not in alignment with nature. Your genes have not yet adapted to eating so often and having to spend so many resources digesting food. Anything that you can do to reduce the workload of your digestive system will further align your body with nature. One mechanism by which this happens is that the detox systems are slowed down during digestion. The less digestion going on, the better your body copes with the toxin overload that day. This benefit is cumulative over time. You will need to do a detox program less often and for a shorter period of time in the years to come. You can replace breakfast, lunch, or dinner with a shake long term. Or switch the liquid meal around making it breakfast one day and dinner the next. You may feel the need for a digestive rest at times and have a day or two of just shakes.

Skip Breakfast Often, Especially If the Previous Dinner Was Late or Huge

This will allow better detox time and give you all the benefits of decreasing the time you spend in the feasting state. Breakfast is a habit that is hard to break for many people, but trust me, once you get the hang of it, you will be grateful to use that option.

Fast Intermittently

Use this experience as a jumpstart to a longer-term implementation of Intermittent Fasting. If you are new to it, this week was a good example of how it feels to fast for twenty-four hours every now and then (as you did between days 4 and 5).

See a Functional Medicine or an Ayurvedic Medicine Doctor

If you resonated with either Functional Medicine (FM) or Ayurvedic Medicine (AM), you can take it a step further and see a practitioner of either, or both. They complement each other beautifully. The Elimination Diet is a tool that comes from the FM world. If you had unexpected symptoms appear while you were detoxing, it is very likely that you have an undetected health issue that your body had adapted to and contributed to your milder symptoms. A good FM or AM practitioner can help you detect the root of the problem.

Use Ayurvedic Herbs

Periodically, regardless of which plan you are following or which lifestyle you choose or go back to after CLEAN7, periodic detox is necessary in today's industrialized urban life. Everyone needs it.

Some more, some less, but everyone needs to support their detox organs. Everyone is exposed and everyone has a backlog of detox tasks that needs to be addressed. The hope is that as time goes by, humankind finds the way to end this dilemma, and detox programs will not be needed anymore. I am afraid, however, that we will need to use this knowledge for at least a few more generations. Choose a lifestyle. Maybe you are one of the people who did the CLEAN7 program as a starting point into wellness. You are now mentally clearer and physically more prepared to make a choice and stick to it. You've been looking for a lifestyle and you are ready to choose. Most experts in the different lifestyles can give you arguments that make so much sense that you want to do what they advise. It is great to know where the advice is coming from and a bit of how the lifestyle you are about to choose came to be. Paleo, vegetarianism, veganism, Atkins, keto, and Eat Right 4 Your Type all have interesting stories, which may help you choose the one, or what version of it, that aligns with your goals.

Detox Your Life

Your Air

According to the watchdog organization the Environment Working Group, the air inside the typical home air is anywhere from two to three times more polluted than outside air. Breathing your hairspray may be more hazardous than second-hand smoke. Anything that has a scent likely contains a chemical that mimics a natural scent rather than a natural source. As long as you can smell any of these products in your house (or your car), they are still off-gassing. Any scent that triggers a headache is a signal that your cells are being disturbed and you should avoid the source of the odor. Inhaling chemicals can be as dangerous as consuming them. With every breath you take, air rushes down your trachea and into your lungs, until it hits the wall of alveoli, the tiny air sacs that grab and absorb that precious commodity: oxygen. Unfortunately, oxygen is not all that is been inhaled. After entering the lungs, molecules of toxins enter the bloodstream and circulate throughout the body.

The contemporary household is a virtual chemistry lab of airborne toxins. Fumes off-gas from paint, upholstery foam, fabric finishes, wood floor sealants and furniture glues, synthetic carpeting, and more. Vinyl flooring is particularly toxic, as polyvinyl chloride

(PVC) off-gasses for years after installation. PBDEs (polybrominated diphenyl ethers), which can cause neurological and developmental damage in infants and children, are found in fire retardants, as well as computers, TV sets, cars, and furniture. If you live in new building or have just done some substantial remodeling, construction materials such as PVC pipes, foam insulation, are likely still off-gassing. Reducing exposure to toxins is what green architecture is all about. Another toxin, although not a man-made one, common in certain parts of the country is mold, which also can make its way into your body via inhalation. If you see evidence of mold or suspect you have it, it is critical to deal with it before it damages your health.

Eliminate Offenders

How do you protect yourself from this toxic assault? Obviously, it cannot be done in a day. The first step is to toss out products such as chemical air fresheners, hair spray, and cleaning products filled with chemicals (more on cleaning products, see page 17). Open your windows, weather permitting, to admit fresh air and reduce the burden of indoor air; use your exhaust fan when cooking and in bathrooms without a window; and vacuum and change the filters on your heating/AC systems regularly.

Purify Your Air

The next step would be to look into purchasing an air purifier. Portable units are designed for a single room, but typically are light enough to move from room to room. A whole-house air purifier hooks up to your furnace or ductwork and is best installed when building a house, doing a major remodel, or replacing an old furnace. When shopping for a room unit, consider whether a model has expensive filters that need to be replaced regularly or ones that can be washed. Most units have more than one filter to catch particles of various sizes. Some units have a HEPA filter, which eliminates airborne particles invisible to the naked eye. This is typically the primary filter in portable air purifiers. Some units ionize the air, which creates ozone that can irritate the lungs. Some purifiers kill germs and bacteria more effectively than others. Some use carbon filtration to remove large particles. A little research goes a long way.

Your Water

In chapter 1 you learned already that your city-supplied water is dangerous. The problem of dirty city water is not just something that happened in Flint, Michigan. To a lesser degree, it is in your home as well. Do a quick Google search and see what is going on right now. Even better, get a water expert to test what is flowing from your faucet. Either www.watercheck.com or www.oxygenozone.com can advise you

I've been lucky to learn about different things from real masters, such as when I sat with Dr. Narendra for weeks and learned about Ayurveda. I learned about water from another master, William Wendling. Growing up in a farm, William loved to wander off on his own into the forest. His favorite hideout was a natural spring where he would drink and bathe in the water. He noticed early on that the spring water tasted and felt so much better than the water from the well next to his house, and he became somewhat obsessed with understanding why. When he was in his late teens, his father died, and an autopsy showed hardened arteries and kidney stones. William had just finished reading the book *The Shocking Truth About Water* by Paul Bragg and became convinced that his farm's well water had something to do with the autopsy findings. He soon learned enough to test water himself and found that the well water was hard water, meaning it contained certain hard minerals, such as magnesium and calcium carbonates. His obsession with understanding water became a mission to find the best way to purify the water for homes and families like his. After years of meticulous research, he designed the best water systems for whole houses, drinking/cooking water in the kitchen, and even for swimming pools. William's vision was to transform city-supplied water into a version most like his childhood natural spring water and have it flow from every faucet in the house. These are the crucially important multiple steps that he included in his filter designs, which are the ones you should look for when you buy a water filtration system:

1. *Carbon filtration* removes all dirt that can be seen in the form of sediment and debris. Granular carbon is okay but solid blocks are better since they remove smaller particles and VOCs (volatile organic contaminants). Carbon blocks are especially important in the kitchen units to remove heavy metals, and improve smell and taste.

2. *Reverse osmosis membrane* is the step William calls "fresh squeezing your own pure water," since this is exactly what happens across a reverse osmosis (RO) membrane: pure water squeezes through and dirty water is diverted for disposal. The membrane also removes the water's hardness in the form of calcium and magnesium carbonates, bringing the water to 85-to 90-percent pure.

3. *Mixed bed deionization* involves having water flow through electrically charged resin beads after the RO membrane captures more impurities and further purifies water.

4. *Remineralization and alkalization* is achieved with an in-line filter with marine-grade coral calcium sand, containing more than seventy naturally occurring trace minerals. This process mimics what the water in his childhood natural spring passed through.

5. *A coconut carbon filter* is the final addition to make the water taste as natural as possible.

I have been using William's filters for more than ten years and I still get excited when he stops to visit and brings all the latest devices to better purify water. He has also made my swimming pool chlorine free, which people notice, finding that their skin is soft after swimming, as though they had just applied moisturizer.

If your budget does not allow for a sophisticated system such as the one described above, do whatever you can. Don't buy water in plastic bottles. Get a pitcher filter with carbon filter for your drinking water. There are all kinds of filters you can get, under the sink, on-counter, and faucet mounted. Use the list of steps I described above to ask your salesperson how it compares to whatever you are considering buying.

For more info on water filtration systems go to www.oxygen ozone.com

For more links to resources on cleaning and detoxing your home, room by room, visit www.cleanprogram.com/clean7.

The CLEAN7 Kitchen and Recipes

Introduction to the CLEAN7 Recipes

By Chef James Barry

I met Dr. Junger more than twelve years ago while cooking dinner for the CLEAN team at their then-headquarters in Los Angeles. I'll never forget that night because Alejandro did something that has never happened before or since in my career as a chef: he asked me to sit down and join the group for dinner. We've been friends ever since.

I'm overjoyed to have been invited to contribute my recipes to CLEAN7. Besides sharing a similar view of food as medicine, Alejandro and I also believe that the energy you put into making food is the energy you receive when you eat it. We are what we eat, yet your constitution—or dosha—informs each of us *what* we should eat.

Find Your Dosha

Combining the more than 5,000-year-old Ayurvedic culinary practices with the CLEAN7 program principles has been an exciting challenge. In the following recipe section, you'll find seven shakes plus seven meals that can also serve as snacks for each of the three doshas. Once you've identified your most dominant dosha (see the Find Your Dosha Questionnaire on page 156), choose your recipes from that section.

Ingredients and Soaking

Some of the recipes may seem unfamiliar at first but know that I've designed them to be as simple to make as possible. Others, such as quinoa tabouleh, may be familiar but some of the ingredients likely differ from those to which you are accustomed. If you cannot find certain ingredients locally, you may need to order them online.

We follow proper soaking and cooking practices for legumes (beans and lentils), grains, nuts, and seeds. Why? Soaking reduces cook time, supports the breakdown of phytic acid, and supports proper digestion. The minimum soaking time for each such recipe is indicated, as is the active prep and cook time. The best approach is to presoak any items overnight. Then drain the water (in most cases) and use the ingredients per the recipe instructions. Some recipes call for soaking flax meal or chia seeds, which can be done in a matter of minutes.

The Right Stuff: Countertop Appliances

A high-speed blender is essential to make the shakes that are integral to the CLEAN7 program. Two other optional appliances are great time savers. Using a food processor or pressure cooker (or an instant pot) whenever possible will shorten your time in the kitchen and make cooking a lot easier.

- **A blender** should have several settings and a motor powerful enough to handle frozen fruit and ice cubes. Some of the soup recipes also call for a blender. Remember, liquid meals are effectively predigested, making them ideal for the program. My Vitamix is also capable of making nut butters, among many other culinary chores, but Hamilton Beach, Cuisinart, and Panasonic also make powerful models, which can run you $400 to $500. If you plan to use your blender primarily for making shakes, smoothies, and pureed soups, you could get away with a less expensive and less powerful model. Stanley Black & Decker, Waring, and Cuisinart make machines that cost between $50 to $100. An alternative is the so-called personal blender, which comes with one or more "to go" mixing containers. Another advantage of a personal blender is that you are likely to use it more often, particularly if you live alone. It is also easier to clean and whip up single portions than a larger blender. I recommend the NutriBullet Pro, which can also crush ice. Brands such as Magic Bullet, BlendJet, Stanley Black & Decker, Keemo, and Chulux are other options. If this is your only blender be sure to get one with at least a 900-watt motor to do more than just make shakes.

- **A multi-cooker,** aka a quick cooker, may be the new kid on the counter, but it is no fad. It lives up to both its names, saving you time and eliminating the mess and odors involved in certain jobs previously handled by your cooktop or oven. This ambidextrous appliance handles the functions that once required a slow-cooker (aka a Crock-Pot), rice cooker, pressure cooker, steamer, warming pot, yogurt maker, and grill. It quickly cooks rice, pressure-cooks legumes, and sautés vegetables, making it particularly useful for Ayurvedic recipes. Highly rated brands include Breville, Gourmia, Instant Pot, Philips, and T-fal. Prices range considerably, depending upon size and programming features, from about $80 for a three-quart model without auto-programmable features to more than $300 for a nine-quart model with all the bells and whistles. Most brands come in three-, six-, and eight-quart models. Pick one that best fits your family size or how often you cook for a crowd. Not all pots perform every function listed above, so make sure they match to your current cooking style or functions you plan to use in the future. Some models allow you to preprogram them or even hook them up to Alexa. Others require you to set features such as cook time and temperature.

- **A food processor** does almost all the prep work your grandma used to do by hand: chopping, grating, grinding, slicing, mincing, and pureeing. It's also a great time and money saver. Make your own guacamole, hummus, and salad dressing in a matter of minutes for less money than commercial versions—minus additives, preservatives, and other suspect ingredients. Although you won't be eating cheese or eggs this week, a food processor also grates block cheese in a matter of seconds and whips up mayo made with extra virgin olive oil or avocado oil. A number of the dishes, such as Fakora and Bella Bites in the recipe section, call for a food processor. Mini processors are great for chopping a small handful of nuts, a bunch of parsley, or a single onion, but a full-size model can handle pretty much any job you throw at it. A 500- to 600-watt motor can handle most jobs but look for a heavy-duty model with a motor of 700 watts or higher if you plan to knead dough or grind meat. The number of servings you typically make should determine bowl size. If it is rarely more than four, a nine-cup bowl should be sufficient, but if you usually cook for a crowd or freeze portions for later use, opt for an eleven- to fourteen-cup model. A three-cup bowl is usually sufficient for single or double portions. A maximum liquid line helps avoid messy overflow. A wide chute enables you to add large pieces of food to the bowl while the processor is running, so you need to spend less time prepping ingredients.

A pulse button helps avoid over processing. Levers and buttons are easy to operate but can trap spills, making a touchpad worth the added cost. A metal S-blade for mincing, chopping, and pureeing and two others to slice and grate are standard. Stainless steel blades perform best. Kneading bread requires a plastic blade. Food processors start at about $50 and go all the way up to $350, depending upon brand, bowl size, wattage, and added features. Breville, Hamilton Beach, Cuisinart, and KitchenAid are all excellent brands.

Suit Your Eating Style and Dietary Preferences

Before beginning the CLEAN7 program, pick the shakes and meals that most appeal to you. Snacks are not mandatory, but if you feel you must have something between a breakfast shake and lunch or between lunch and your evening shake, you can always have a half portion of a meal as a snack. Certain days call for a snack *instead* of a meal. Again, have a half portion of a meal recipe or another snack that complies with the Elimination Diet and your dosha guidelines. Refer to the CLEAN7 Week's Protocol (page 145) for details.

If you're Vata or Kapha dominant, you'll want to serve all your shakes, meals, and snacks lightly heated or at room temperature. Since all recipes are for two or occasionally more servings, you'll inevitably have leftovers unless your partner is doing the program with you. We recommend eating leftovers the following day unless you're on the fasting day of the detox. Here are two quick tricks to reheating food without using a microwave:

For dry heat, preheat the oven with the baking tray in it. Once the oven has reached the desired temperature, pull out the hot tray with oven mitts, place the food on it, and return to the oven. Your food will be warm within five minutes or less.

For wet heat, place the food to be reheated in a pan or pot with one tablespoon of water. Place on the stovetop over medium heat and cover. The food should be warm within three minutes.

Some of the seven meals are based on animal protein and others rely on plant protein. Half portions of the meals may be eaten as snacks, if you find you need a snack. You'll find that a few meal recipes call for a dosha-appropriate vegetable side dish; others serve as one-dish meals. My hope is that among the seven meal and snack recipes, you'll find several recipes that fit your dietary preferences.

Food Quality Is Always Key

While we don't specify it in the recipes, we recommend that you purchase certified organic fruits and vegetables. Or purchase produce at your local farmers' market where you can ask the farmer how the food has been grown. (It has likely also been just picked that morning or the night before.) We recommend that all animal protein be pasture raised or grass fed and that all fish be wild or sustainably raised. If you must purchase farmed fish, ask your fishmonger what the fish have been fed. Stay away from farmed fish that are fed soy or other grains or contain added color.

Ideally, nuts and seeds should be raw and unsalted. The next best option is roasted and unsalted nuts and seeds.

Beans and lentils are best cooked from scratch, which is why we recommend using a pressure cooker. However, we know that sometimes buying canned legumes is a more realistic option. For any canned product, make sure to buy organic and to read the ingredients list. Look for as few ingredients as possible and only ingredients you recognize. Choose canned beans, for example, with only beans, water, and kombu (a seaweed that aids digestibility). Use canned coconut milk with just two ingredients, water and coconut. Pass on any product with added sugar in any form. Apply these label rules to any premade or packaged item you buy.

We recommend buying whole spices and using a designated spice grinder or mortar and pestle to grind them. Ground spices spoil quickly and lose their potency over time. You'll note that when a recipe calls for spices, they are first cooked briefly in some oil or a dry pan. This revives the spice and brings out the fragrance.

For salt, we recommend sea salt or pink Himalayan salt. Another effective option, but one that is harder to find, is black salt, which is mined in soft-stone quarries in India. Rich in minerals and with a smoky, sulfurous aroma, black salt does not increase the sodium content in blood so it is recommended for people who are Kapha dominant. Black salt can be found in Indian markets or online.

If you can't find certain ingredients locally, check online. If that isn't an option, review your Dosha Food List (page 158) and pick an item that is closest to what you can find at your local grocery store.

Sustain the Benefits of CLEAN7

As you transition off any cleanse, it can be a challenge to maintain the good habits you've recently brought to your day-to-day routine. To support your process, I've provided you with a complete day of clean eating—actually more, since you have a choice between a shake and a breakfast dish. The seven Celebratory Meals that start on page 272 comply with the Elimination Diet. All prove that there is no need to deprive yourself of great-tasting food while eating healthy foods. Eating the CLEAN7 way needn't be the exception. It can be a part of your everyday food choices.

I hope you enjoy these recipes. Thank you for letting me into your kitchen. I'm grateful to have contributed to your health journey!

Cheers,

Chef James

Vata Recipes

Shakes

All shake recipes are for two portions. Unless you are doing CLEAN7 with a partner, you can refrigerate one portion and have the other half in the evening or late afternoon. However, vata constitutions should avoid ice cold drinks (and cold foods) so let them come to room temperature after removing from the fridge. Use room-temperature filtered water, coconut water, or unsweetened almond or cashew milk. Most of the shakes require you soak seeds, nuts, or legumes for at least six hours or overnight. Get in the habit of putting them out to soak before you go to bed. However, the Black Forest Shake requires no soaking and the Island Strong and Salud Shakes need just ten minutes of soaking.

Island Strong Shake

SERVES: 2

SOAK TIME: 10 minutes

PREP TIME: 5 minutes

Inspired by the mango lassi drink that is a staple of Indian restaurants, my dairy-free twist uses coconut milk. Lime juice and zest brighten the mango flavor. Use canned coconut milk, not the beverage in a carton. Avoid coconut milk with guar gum in the ingredients list.

16 ounces unsweetened coconut milk

1 tablespoon chia seeds

1 cup frozen or fresh mango

½ teaspoon lime juice

Pinch of lime zest

½ teaspoon fresh, grated ginger

1 tablespoon coconut or MCT oil

1 micro-spoon powdered stevia, 2 drops liquid stevia, or 1 teaspoon
    coconut nectar

Pinch of sea salt or pink Himalayan salt

Soak the chia seeds in a bowl with the coconut milk for 10 minutes or until the seeds are soft. Set aside without draining.

Add the coconut milk and chia seeds, mango, lime juice, lime zest, fresh ginger, coconut oil, stevia, and salt to a high-speed blender. Blend until smooth. If you used frozen mango, allow the shake to reach room temperature prior to drinking.

To serve, pour into two glasses.

Soother Shake

SERVES: 2

SOAK TIME: 6 hours or overnight

PREP TIME: 5 minutes

There's something incredibly soothing about pecans. Their natural sweetness is both warming and light. Add tahini (pureed sesame seeds) and almonds and you'll have something extra special.

½ cup pecan halves

2 cups filtered water

1 tablespoon chia seeds

2 cups unsweetened almond milk

2 tablespoons tahini

¼ teaspoon cinnamon

¼ teaspoon cardamom powder (optional)

½ teaspoon alcohol-free vanilla extract or vanilla powder
   (ground vanilla bean)

1 micro-spoon powdered stevia, 2 drops of liquid stevia,
   or 1 teaspoon coconut nectar

¼ cup prune juice (100 percent juice, not from concentrate)

1 tablespoon lemon juice

Pinch of sea salt or pink Himalayan salt

In a medium-size bowl, soak the pecans in 2 cups of filtered water for a minimum of 6 hours or overnight. Drain and set almonds aside.

Soak the chia seeds in a small bowl with the almond milk for 10 minutes or until the seeds are soft. Set aside without draining.

Add the almond milk, chia seeds, drained pecans, tahini, cinnamon, optional cardamom, vanilla extract, stevia, prune juice, lemon juice, and salt to a high-speed blender. Blend until smooth.

Allow to reach room temperature before drinking.

To serve, pour into two glasses.

Tiger's Milk Shake

SERVES: 2
SOAK TIME: 24 hours
PREP TIME: 5 minutes

This is my take on horchata, a Latin grain-based drink also known as the Gods' Nectar. Tiger nuts are not actually nuts, but tubers with a sweet taste reminiscent of coconut. Tiger nuts require a longer soaking time than other recipes. If you can't find them, substitute almonds or almond butter.

¼ cup peeled tiger nuts or 1 tablespoon unsweetened almond
   butter
2¾ cups filtered water, divided
3 dates, pitted
1 tablespoon chia seeds
1 cup unsweetened almond or cashew milk
¼ cup cooked basmati rice
½ teaspoon cinnamon
½ teaspoon alcohol-free vanilla extract or vanilla powder
   (ground vanilla bean)
Pinch of sea salt or pink Himalayan salt
Pinch of cardamom powder (optional)
Pinch of ginger powder (optional)
Pinch turmeric powder (optional)

In a medium-size bowl, soak the tiger nuts in 2 cups of filtered water for a minimum of 24 hours. Drain and set the nuts aside.

Soak the dates in a small bowl of warm water for 10 minutes or until soft. Drain water and set aside.

Soak the chia seeds in a small bowl with the almond or cashew milk for 10 minutes or until the seeds are soft. Set the nut milk and seeds aside until ready to use.

Add the soaked chia seeds and nut milk, soaked tiger nuts, soaked dates, basmati rice, remaining ¾ cup of filtered water, cinnamon, vanilla extract, and salt, along with the optional cardamom, ginger, and turmeric to a high-speed blender. Blend until smooth.

Allow to reach room temperature before pouring into two glasses.

Berry Blast Shake

SERVES: 2
SOAK TIME: 10 minutes
PREP TIME: 5 minutes

Berries are flavorful without being too sweet—or at least as sweet as many other fruits. The only berry that is off limits during the cleanse is strawberry. Otherwise, choose the mix of berries you most enjoy.

¼ cup hulled sunflower seeds
1½ cups filtered water, divided
1 tablespoon chia seeds
10 ounces unsweetened almond milk
1 cup mixed fresh or frozen berries (raspberries, blueberries, or blackberries)
½ cup raw spinach
1 tablespoon lemon juice
½ teaspoon fresh grated ginger
2 micro-spoons powdered stevia or 2 drops liquid stevia

Presoak the sunflower seeds in 1 cup of filtered water for a minimum of 6 hours or overnight. Drain and set aside.

Soak the chia seeds in a bowl with the almond milk for 10 minutes or until the seeds are soft. Set the seeds and almond milk aside until ready to use.

Place the soaked sunflower seeds, chia seeds in almond milk, berries, spinach, ½ cup of water, lemon juice, grated ginger, and stevia in a high-speed blender. Blend until smooth.

If you used frozen berries, allow the shake to come to room temperature before pouring into two glasses.

Black Forest Shake

SERVES: 2

PREP TIME: 5 minutes

When you need a chocolate fix, make this shake. Processed chocolate full of sugar is not supported in Ayurveda, but raw cacao powder is. A hint of cherry and satiating healthy fat will blunt your cravings and leave you feeling satisfyingly full. This shake requires no presoaking, making it handy for mornings on the run.

2 cups unsweetened almond milk
1 tablespoon raw cacao powder
½ cup frozen cherries (about 10 cherries)
¼ cup cooked yam, peeled*
1 tablespoon coconut oil or MCT oil
1 micro-spoon powdered stevia, 2 drops liquid stevia,
    or 1 tablespoon coconut nectar
Pinch of sea salt or pink Himalayan salt

Place the almond milk, cacao powder, cherries, yam, coconut oil, stevia, and salt in a high-speed blender. Blend until smooth. Allow to come to room temperature prior to drinking.

To serve, pour into two glasses.

* For a quick, cooked yam, steam a whole yam in a covered pot over water on high for 10 minutes. Once it cools, peel the yam and measure out the amount needed for the recipe. Save the remaining yam for another meal.

Detoxifier Shake

SERVES: 2

SOAK TIME: 6 hours or overnight

PREP TIME: 5 minutes

COOK TIME: 35 minutes (using a multi-cooker)

Mung (or moong) beans are tridoshic, meaning they are balancing to all three doshas. Mung beans are a powerful tool for detoxing and also support an increased metabolism. This mild, warm drink is like a soup. Make sure to drink lots of water throughout the day after having this shake.

½ cup green mung beans

4 cups filtered water plus more for soaking

1 teaspoon coconut oil

½ teaspoon cumin seeds

¼ teaspoon fennel seeds

¼ teaspoon turmeric powder

¼ teaspoon coriander powder

2 tablespoons lemon juice

¼ teaspoon sea salt or pink Himalayan salt

In a medium-size bowl, soak the mung beans in enough water (about 2 cups) to cover and allow room for expansion. Soak for a minimum of 6 hours or overnight. Drain and set aside.

On the stove top: Place a medium-size sauce pot over medium heat and add the coconut oil. When it has heated, add the cumin, fennel, turmeric, and coriander. Allow to cook for 1 minute or until fragrant. Add the soaked mung beans and 4 cups of filtered water. Bring to a boil, then lower the temperature, cover the pot and simmer until cooked, approximately 2 hours.

In a multi-cooker: Set pot to Sauté. Add the coconut oil and heat. Add the cumin, fennel, turmeric, and coriander. Allow to cook for 1 minute or until fragrant. Add soaked mung beans and 4 cups of filtered water. Press Cancel. Cover the pot with the lid, press the

Bean button (or set it for 30 minutes). The unit will ding when the meal is ready.

Uncover the pot, pour the entire pot of beans and liquid into an appropriate-size high-speed blender. Add the salt and 1 tablespoon lemon juice and secure the lid. As a precaution, place a folded towel over the blender lid before turning on the unit. Hot liquids have a tendency to spit up to the lid and could burn your hand. With the towel in place, blend until the mixture forms a smooth soup. Taste and add more lemon juice if you want a brighter flavor.

To serve, pour into two mugs.

Salud Shake

SERVES: 2
SOAK TIME: 10 minutes
PREP TIME: 10 minutes

This shake maximizes the nutritional value of green vegetables with omega-3 fatty acids in the form of chia seeds. Think of it as like drinking a salad with a really healthy dressing. Start your day with this shake and you'll feel energized and clear headed.

1 tablespoon chia seeds
5 ounces coconut water
3-inch piece peeled cucumber
1 small head of romaine lettuce, about 2 cups
½ cup packed spinach
¼ cup packed parsley leaves, thick stems removed
½ avocado, peel removed
1 small green apple, peeled and cored
2 tablespoons lime juice
7 ounces filtered water
1 micro-spoon powdered stevia or 2 drops liquid stevia
Pinch of sea salt or pink Himalayan salt

Soak the chia seeds in a small bowl in the coconut water for 10 minutes or until the seeds are soft. Set aside without draining.

While the chia seeds are soaking, prep the cucumber, romaine lettuce, spinach, parsley, and avocado.

In a small pot over high heat, steam the green apple over water until soft (about 2 minutes). Drain and set aside.

Add the chia seeds–coconut water mixture, cucumber, romaine lettuce, spinach, parsley, avocado, steamed apple, lime juice, filtered water, stevia, and salt to a high-speed blender. Blend until smooth. Add additional water if you like a more liquid beverage.

To serve, pour into two glasses and drink at room temperature.

Vata Meals and Snacks

Several of the vata recipes require you to soak seeds, nuts, or legumes for at least 6 hours or overnight. Get in the habit of putting them to soak them the night before you make a recipe. Most recipes are for two meal portions, but if you are having one as a snack (or light meal) instead, typically you will have four snack portions. Each recipe provides the number of portions for both a meal and a snack. Unless you are doing CLEAN7 with a partner, you can have one meal portion and refrigerate the other half for the following day. Some meals require a vata-acceptable vegetable side dish to complete the meal. If you make a recipe as a snack, you will usually have three snack portions to refrigerate or freeze for another time. Being vata dominant, you'll want to ensure that all meals and snacks are warm or at room temperature before serving.

Chickpea Street Tacos

SERVES: 2 (2 TACOS) AS A MEAL
SERVES: 4 (1 TACO) AS A SNACK
PREP TIME: 10 minutes
COOK TIME: 20 minutes

You won't miss the corn with these delicious tacos. The chickpea pancake folds like a soft taco. Chimichurri, a flavorful Latin herb sauce, replaces salsa. You might find you like it so much that you'll want to put it on everything!

½ cup chickpea flour
½ cup filtered water
¼ teaspoon sea salt or pink Himalayan salt
¼ teaspoon baking soda
1 teaspoon minced green onion (green part only)
1 tablespoon avocado oil, divided
6 to 8 ounces chicken breast or thigh, diced*
1 clove garlic, thinly sliced
1 red radish, thinly sliced
¼ cup chopped zucchini
¼ cup chopped yellow squash
½ cup spinach
1 avocado, sliced
1 teaspoon nutritional yeast flakes (optional)

FOR THE CHIMICHURRI SAUCE
1 green onion, roughly chopped
½ cup Italian parsley, thick stems removed
¼ cup cilantro, thick stems removed
1 shallot (about the size of a tablespoon),
    peeled and roughly chopped
¼ cup lemon juice
¼ cup extra-virgin olive oil
¼ teaspoon sea salt or pink Himalayan salt (or to taste)

In a medium-size bowl, whisk the chickpea flour, filtered water, salt, baking soda, and minced green onion until smooth. Set aside.

In a large skillet over medium heat, heat 2 teaspoons of avocado oil. Add the chicken and garlic and allow to brown, about 3 minutes, turning midway. Add the radish, zucchini, yellow squash, and spinach. Cook 2 more minutes, making sure chicken is fully cooked. Remove from burner, cover, and set aside.

Make the chimichurri sauce: Place the green onion, parsley, cilantro, shallot, and lemon juice in the bowl of a food processor and pulse until well minced. Drizzle the extra-virgin olive oil through the chute while the processor is running until well incorporated. Using a flexible spatula, scrape the mixture into a small bowl. Mix in the salt and set aside.

Place a large cast-iron pan over medium heat on the cooktop. Add a teaspoon of avocado oil. Once a drop of water sizzles in the pan, scoop ¼ cup of the chickpea batter into the pan, spreading the mix until it is the size of a small tortilla. Cook until you see little bubbles forming on the top, about 30 to 40 seconds, then, using a thin spatula, flip the "tortilla" and cook for another 30 to 40 seconds. Remove from the skillet and place on a plate. Repeat three more times.

For a meal, place two tortillas on each plate. Distribute the avocado slices evenly over the tortillas and top with the chicken and vegetables mixture in four equal portions. Drizzle ½ teaspoon of the chimichurri sauce over each taco and sprinkle with an optional pinch of nutritional yeast.

For a snack, have only one tortilla.

Refrigerate leftover chicken and vegetables in a container with a lid. Place a piece of parchment paper between each tortilla, place in a lidded container, and refrigerate.

* Use free-range or pasture-raised chicken.

Kitchari

SERVES: 2 AS A MEAL

SERVES: 4 AS A SNACK

SOAK TIME: 6 hours or overnight

PREP TIME: 7 minutes

COOK TIME: 30 minutes (in a multi-cooker)

The ultimate Ayurvedic detox meal, this dish is tridoshic, means it is suitable for all three doshas. Yellow mung (moong) dal is a delicate legume that cooks quickly and is easy to digest. If you can't find it at your local store, it is readily available on online.

¼ cup yellow mung dal

¼ cup basmati rice

2 cups filtered water, plus more for soaking

2 tablespoons coconut oil

1 small white or yellow onion

1 small zucchini

1 small carrot

½ teaspoon cumin seeds

¼ teaspoon black mustard seeds

¼ teaspoon ground turmeric

¼ teaspoon ground coriander

½ teaspoon sea salt or pink Himalayan salt

1 tablespoon lemon or lime juice

Cilantro, for garnish (optional)

In a medium-size bowl, combine the mung dal and basmati rice with enough filtered water to cover. Allow to soak for a minimum of 6 hours or overnight. Strain in a mesh strainer and set aside.

Add the onion, zucchini, and carrot to the bowl of a food processor. Pulse until finely chopped.

On the stove top: Place a small pot over medium heat. Add the coconut oil and heat. Add the mix of onion, zucchini, and carrot along with the cumin, black mustard seed, turmeric, and coriander. Allow to cook for 1 to 2 minutes. Then add the dal and rice mixture and 2 cups of filtered water. Bring to a boil, then lower the temperature, cover the pot, and simmer until cooked, approximately 2 hours.

In a multi-cooker: Set the pot to Sauté. Add the coconut oil and allow it to heat. Add the vegetable mix, cumin, black mustard, turmeric, and coriander. Allow to cook for 1 to 2 minutes. Add the dal and rice mixture and 2 cups of water. Press Cancel. Place the lid on the pot, press the Bean button (or set it for 30 minutes). The pot will ding when the meal is ready.

Once cooked by either method, uncover, add salt and lemon juice and gently mix until evenly incorporated.

For a meal, divide the mixture into two bowls. Sprinkle with optional minced cilantro and serve.

For a snack, have a half bowl, top with the optional cilantro, and refrigerate the rest.

Waffle Hash Open-Face Sandwich

SERVES: 2 (2 TOASTS) AS A MEAL

SERVES: 4 (1 TOAST) AS A SNACK

SOAK TIME: 10 minutes

PREP TIME: 10 minutes

COOK TIME: 10 minutes

A healthier version of avocado toast, this recipe is easiest to make with a waffle iron, but if you don't have one, just make them as you would a pancake. The flax meal provides the binding you would normally get from an egg.

1 tablespoon flax meal

2 tablespoons warm filtered water

1 sweet potato, grated or noodled (using a spiralizer)

1 small onion, peeled and sliced

3 tablespoons brown rice flour

1 tablespoon arrowroot

3 tablespoons black, white, or mixed sesame seeds

½ teaspoon sea salt or pink Himalayan salt

1 tablespoon coconut oil, melted

Avocado or sunflower oil cooking spray

8 asparagus spears, sliced in half lengthwise.

2 red radishes, thinly sliced

1 avocado, peeled and mashed with a squeeze of lemon and pinch of salt

4 slices (2 ounces each) cooked free-range chicken breast*
   (or 6–8 ounces cooked wild-caught salmon)

1 scallion, minced (optional)

Ground black pepper, to taste

In a small cup or bowl, combine the flax meal with 2 tablespoons of filtered water. Set aside to soak for about 10 minutes.

Place the sweet potatoes and onions in a large bowl with the brown rice flour, arrowroot, sesame seeds, salt, and melted coconut oil. Mix until well combined. Add the presoaked flax meal and mix well.

Turn the waffle iron to the highest setting per the instruction manual. Once ready, mist the waffle iron with avocado or sunflower oil. Add ⅓ cup of the sweet potato mix to the waffle iron, carefully spreading the mixture so that a thin layer fills the waffle cavity. Close the lid and cook for 5 minutes. The waffle iron may indicate it's ready before that time, but allow the sweet potato mixture to cook as close to 5 minutes as possible without burning. Once crisp, set the waffles aside on a cooling rack and keep them warm in a low oven. Repeat until all the batter is used.

Discard the fibrous ends of the asparagus and cut the spears so they are the length of the waffles. Steam the asparagus and radishes over boiling water for 1 to 2 minutes, or until they are soft but not mushy. Drain and set aside.

To serve, spread equal amounts of the mashed avocado over the four hash toasts. Layer on equal amounts of the asparagus and radish. Place two chicken rolls (or pieces of salmon) on top of each toast. Garnish with a dash of black pepper and a pinch of minced scallion.

As a snack, prepare as above but have only one hash toast instead of two.

* Use free-range or pasture-raised chicken or wild-caught salmon.

Tur-Veggie Patty

SERVES: 4 (1 PATTY) AS A MEAL
SERVES: 8 (1 SMALL PATTY) AS A SNACK
SOAK TIME: 6 hours or overnight
PREP TIME: 10 minutes
COOK TIME: 10 minutes

My favorite way to eat a ground patty is with loads of veggies mixed in. Besides tasting great, this is also a fantastic way to get more vegetables into your diet. This turkey-veggie mix can be stored in a refrigerator for up to five days or in the freezer for two weeks, making it particularly handy when you have little time to prepare a meal from scratch.

¼ cup walnuts or pecans
2 cups filtered water
2 peeled shallots, divided
1 small zucchini, roughly chopped
¼ cup cilantro, thick stems removed
1 carrot, roughly chopped
2 kale leaves, stems removed or 1 packed cup of spinach
½ teaspoon dried oregano
½ teaspoon granulated garlic
¼ teaspoon ground cumin
½ teaspoon sea salt or pink Himalayan salt
1 pound ground dark turkey meat (or ground chicken meat)*
2 tablespoons avocado oil, divided
1 small parsnip, sliced into thin rounds
4 green lettuce leaves
1 avocado, pit removed, sliced

LEMON VINAIGRETTE

¼ cup lemon juice

1 teaspoon tahini

1 tablespoon nutritional yeast flakes

¼ teaspoon sea salt or pink Himalayan salt

¼ teaspoon ground black pepper

¼ teaspoon granulated garlic

1 micro-spoon powdered stevia or 1 drop liquid stevia

½ cup extra-virgin olive oil

Place the walnuts or pecans in a large bowl with 2 cups of water to soak for 6 hours minimum or overnight. Strain, rinse. and set aside until ready to use.

Place the presoaked nuts, 1 shallot, zucchini, cilantro, carrot, kale (or spinach), oregano, granulated garlic, cumin, and salt in a food processor, and pulse until well minced.

In a large bowl, mix the turkey with the minced vegetables until well incorporated. Shape into four same-size patties and place on a baking sheet. (If you are making this recipe as a snack, shape into eight small patties instead.)

In a large frying pan over medium heat, add 1 tablespoon of avocado oil. Once warm, place the patties in the pan and allow to cook until brown, about 3 minutes (2 minutes for smaller patties). Flip and repeat for other side, about 3 minutes (2 minutes for smaller patties) or until the patties are fully cooked.

While the patties are cooking, thinly slice the shallot.

In a smaller frying pan, add a tablespoon of avocado oil, the sliced parsnips, and remaining shallot. Cook until lightly browned on both sides. If the parsnip slices are thick, cook them a little longer. When finished, set aside.

For the dressing: Place the lemon juice, tahini, nutritional yeast flakes, sea salt, ground black pepper, granulated garlic, stevia, and extra-virgin olive oil in a mason jar. Tighten the lid and shake vigorously until well mixed.

To serve as a meal, add a dollop of dressing to each lettuce leaf and top with a patty. Evenly distribute the sliced avocado and top with the cooked parsnips and shallots.

To serve as a snack, as above but with a small patty, half a lettuce leaf, and smaller amount of avocado. Omit the cooked parsnips and shallots.

* Use free-range or pasture-raised turkey or chicken.

Bella Bites

SERVES: 2 AS A MEAL
SERVES: 4 AS A SNACK
PREP TIME: 5 minutes
COOK TIME: 15 minutes

This dish is inspired by the Shake 'n Bake style of cooking that was so popular in the 1970s. This gluten-free version uses seeds instead of bread crumbs to give the chicken a crisp texture. Don't limit this dish to just chicken. You can use a fish such as cod as well! These bites are so packed with flavor that they need no sauce.

Avocado oil spray, for pan
½ cup raw pepitas (pumpkin seeds)
¼ teaspoon powdered sage
¼ teaspoon ground mustard
½ teaspoon dried oregano
½ teaspoon dried thyme
½ teaspoon dried parsley
½ teaspoon granulated onion
½ teaspoon granulated garlic
½ teaspoon sea salt or pink Himalayan salt
1 tablespoon nutritional yeast
8 ounces chicken wings (about 4–6), chicken tenders,
   or cod filets*
1 tablespoon extra-virgin olive oil

Preheat the oven to 400°F. Lightly spray a baking sheet with avocado oil.

Place the raw pepitas, powdered sage, ground mustard, dried oregano, dried thyme, dried parsley, granulated onion, granulated garlic, salt, and nutritional yeast in the bowl of a food processor, and process until very fine. Empty into a medium-size bowl.

If using chicken tenders or cod, cut into bite-size pieces. In a small bowl, toss the protein of choice in with the olive oil. Toss to mix.

Dredge a wing or a couple of pieces of chicken or cod in the bowl of crumbs until both sides are well coated. Place on the greased baking sheet and repeat with the other pieces.

Cook for 5 to 7 minutes. Flip over, using a thin spatula, and cook another 5 to 7 minutes or until fully cooked. The thickness of the chicken or cod will determine the cooking time.

Remove from the oven and allow to cool for 2 to 3 minutes before serving.

For a meal, serve with a portion of vata dosha–appropriate vegetables.

* Use free-range or pasture-raised chicken or sustainable wild-caught fish.

Quinoa Tabouleh

SERVES: 2 AS A MEAL

SERVES: 4 AS A SNACK

SOAK TIME: 1 hour or overnight

PREP TIME: 5 minutes

COOK TIME: 20 minutes

Quinoa (pronounced keen-wah), an ancient grain originally from South America, is high in protein and has a nutty taste. It also makes a great gluten-free substitute for bulgur wheat in this refreshing and filling Levantine-inspired salad.

½ cup uncooked quinoa

¾ cup filtered water plus more for soaking

1 carrot, roughly chopped

1 red radish

1 scallion, roughly chopped

1 bunch cilantro, thick stems removed (about 1 cup)

8 fresh mint leaves

2 tablespoons lemon juice

4 tablespoons extra-virgin olive oil

½ cup diced cucumber

½ cup diced jicama (optional)

½ teaspoon sea salt or pink Himalayan salt

½ teaspoon sumac (optional)

In a medium-size bowl, combine the quinoa with enough filtered water to cover. Allow to soak for a minimum of 1 hour or overnight. Strain through a fine-mesh strainer.

Place the quinoa in a large dry skillet on medium heat to dry it out. Watch the pan closely, stirring the quinoa with a wooden spatula so it doesn't burn, for about 5 minutes.

Put ¾ cup of water in a medium-size pot and bring to a boil. Add the quinoa, cover, and return to a boil. Turn off the heat and keep the pot covered for a minimum of 15 minutes or until all the water has been absorbed.

While the quinoa is cooking, place the carrot, radish, scallion, cilantro, and mint leaves in the bowl of a food processor. Pulse until minced but not mushy.

Empty the warm quinoa into a large bowl. Add the minced vegetables, cucumber, jicama, lemon juice, extra-virgin olive oil, salt, and sumac. Mix until well incorporated and serve.

As a meal, increase the amounts of veggies in the recipe or accompany with a vata-appropriate vegetable side dish.

NOTE: While tabouleh is traditionally eaten cold, individuals with the vata-dominant dosha should eat this recipe warm or at room temperature.

Fakora

SERVES: 2 OR 3 (6 OR 7 PATTIES) AS A MEAL
SERVES: 5 (4 PATTIES EACH) AS A SNACK
PREP TIME: 5 minutes
COOK TIME: 25 minutes

This recipe was inspired by Egyptian and Levantine falafel and the Indian pakora, both of which are usually deep fried. This healthier version is baked instead. It is made with lots of veggies and just a little chickpea flour. I grate the ginger on a zester. Eat the patties dry, or pair them with pesto or chimichurri sauce (page 205).

Avocado oil spray, for pan
2 tablespoons extra-virgin olive oil
1 sweet potato, peeled and roughly chopped
½ cauliflower head, roughly chopped
1 medium onion, thinly sliced
1 teaspoon grated fresh ginger
1 cup chopped spinach
¼ cup chopped cilantro
½ teaspoon ground turmeric
½ teaspoon granulated garlic
½ teaspoon cumin seed
½ teaspoon sumac
1 teaspoon sea salt or pink Himalayan salt
½ teaspoon lemon zest
1½ cups chickpea (garbanzo) flour
¼–½ cup filtered water

Heat the oven to 425°F. Lightly spray a baking sheet with avocado oil.

Place 2 tablespoons of olive oil, the sweet potato, cauliflower, onion, fresh ginger, spinach, cilantro, ground turmeric, granulated garlic, cumin seed, sumac, salt, lemon zest, and chickpea flour in the bowl of a food processor. Pulse until well mixed, but still slightly chunky. If the mix looks too dry, add ¼ cup of filtered water and pulse again. If still too dry, add the other ¼ cup water and pulse again.

Using a tablespoon, scoop out 20 portions, form into patties, and place on the greased baking sheet.

Bake for 10 minutes, then use a spatula to flip over the patties. Spray or brush each piece with more oil and bake another 15 minutes, until golden brown.

Let cool on the baking sheet for 5 minutes before eating. Store the leftover patties in a container with a lid in the refrigerator for up to two weeks or in the freezer for up to two months.

If serving as a meal, add a side dish of vata dosha–appropriate cooked vegetables.

Pitta Recipes

Shakes

All shake recipes are for two portions. Unless you are doing CLEAN7 with a partner, you can refrigerate one portion and have the other half in the evening or late afternoon. Or halve a recipe if you want to try a different shake for dinner. Most of these shakes are based on coconut milk, rice milk, or almond milk. In lieu of 16 ounces of rice milk, you can substitute a ¼ cup cooked basmati rice with 14 ounces of water. Pitta constitutions can have both cool and warm foods so if you like your shakes on the colder side, feel free to add ice cubes to all but the Detoxifier Shake. Most of the shakes require you soak seeds, nuts, or legumes for at least 6 hours or overnight. Get in the habit of putting them out to soak before you go to bed. However, Black Forest Shake requires no soaking and the Island Strong and Salud Shakes need just 10 minutes of soaking.

Island Strong Shake

SERVES: 2

SOAK TIME: 10 minutes

PREP TIME: 5 minutes

Inspired by the mango lassi drink that is a staple of Indian restaurants, my dairy-free twist is to use coconut milk. Lime juice and zest brighten the mango flavor. Use canned coconut milk, not the beverage in a carton. Try to avoid coconut milk with guar gum in the ingredient list.

1 tablespoon flax meal

16 ounces unsweetened coconut milk

1 cup frozen or fresh mango

½ teaspoon lime juice

Pinch of lime zest

½ teaspoon fresh grated ginger

1 tablespoon coconut or MCT oil

1 micro-spoon powdered stevia, 2 drops liquid stevia,
   or 1 teaspoon coconut nectar

Pinch of salt

Soak the flax meal in a bowl with the coconut milk for 10 minutes or until the seeds are soft.

Place the coconut milk-flax meal mixture, mango, lime juice, lime zest, grated ginger, coconut oil, stevia, and salt in a high-speed blender. Blend until smooth.

To serve, pour into two glasses.

Soother Shake

SERVES: 2

SOAK TIME: 6 hours or overnight

PREP TIME: 5 minutes

Sunflowers induce happiness. Maybe that's why I love mixing sunflower seeds in shakes. Soaking the seeds makes them not only more nutritious but also able to blend more smoothly.

½ cup hulled sunflower seeds

2 cups filtered water

1 tablespoon flax meal

2 cups unsweetened almond milk

2 tablespoons canned coconut milk or coconut cream

¼ teaspoon cinnamon

¼ teaspoon cardamom powder (optional)

½ teaspoon alcohol-free vanilla extract or vanilla powder
   (ground vanilla bean)

3 dried dates, pitted or 1 tablespoon coconut nectar

½ cup pomegranate juice (100 percent juice, not from concentrate)

Pinch of sea salt or pink Himalayan salt

In a medium-size bowl, presoak the sunflower seeds in 2 cups of water to cover with room for expansion. Soak for a minimum of 6 hours or overnight. Drain and set the sunflower seeds aside.

Soak the flax meal in the almond milk for 10 minutes or until soft in a small bowl.

When the flax meal is soft, add the almond milk–flax mixture to a high-speed blender, along with the drained sunflower seeds, coconut milk, cinnamon, optional cardamom powder, vanilla extract, dried dates, pomegranate juice, and salt. Blend until smooth.

To serve, pour into two glasses.

Tiger's Milk Shake

SERVES: 2

SOAK TIME: 24 hours

PREP TIME: 5 minutes

This is my take on horchata, a Latin grain-based drink also known as the Gods' Nectar. Tiger nuts are not actually nuts, but rather tubers with a sweet taste reminiscent of coconut. Tiger nuts require a longer soaking time than other recipes. If you can't find them, substitute almonds or almond butter.

¼ cup peeled tiger nuts or 1 tablespoon unsweetened almond butter

2¾ cups filtered water, divided

1 cup unsweetened almond milk

1 tablespoon flax meal

¼ cup cooked basmati rice

3 dates, pitted

½ teaspoon cinnamon

½ teaspoon alcohol-free vanilla extract or vanilla powder (ground vanilla bean)

Pinch of salt

Pinch of cardamom powder (optional)

Pinch of ginger powder (optional)

Pinch turmeric powder (optional)

In a medium-size bowl, soak the tiger nuts in 2 cups of filtered water for a minimum of 24 hours. Drain and set the nuts aside.

Soak the flax meal in a small bowl with the almond milk for 10 minutes or until the seeds are soft. Set the mixture aside until ready to use.

Place the soaked tiger nuts, the soaked flax meal–almond milk mixture, basmati rice, remaining ¾ cup of filtered water, dates, cinnamon, vanilla extract, and salt, along with the optional cardamom, ginger, and turmeric in a high-speed blender. Blend until smooth.

To serve, pour into two glasses.

Berry Blast Shake

SERVES: 2
SOAK TIME: 6 hours or overnight
PREP TIME: 5 minutes

Berries are flavorful without being too sweet—or at least as sweet as many other fruits. The only berry that is off limits during the cleanse is strawberry. Otherwise, choose the mix of berries you most enjoy.

¼ cup hulled sunflower seeds
1½ cups filtered water, divided
10 ounces unsweetened almond milk
1 tablespoon flax meal
1 cup mixed fresh or frozen berries
  (raspberries, blueberries, or blackberries)
½ cup raw spinach
1 tablespoon lime juice
½ teaspoon fresh grated ginger
2 micro-spoons powdered stevia or 2 drops liquid stevia

Soak the sunflower seeds in 1 cup of filtered water for a minimum of 6 hours or overnight. Drain and set the seeds aside.

Soak the flax meal in a bowl with the almond milk for 10 minutes until soft. Set the mixture aside.

Place the soaked sunflower seeds, flax meal in almond milk, berries, spinach, lime juice, grated ginger, and stevia in a high-speed blender. Blend until smooth.

To serve, pour into two glasses.

Black Forest Shake

SERVES: 2

PREP TIME: 5 minutes

When you need a chocolate fix, make this shake. Processed chocolate full of sugar is not supported in Ayurveda, but raw cacao powder is. A hint of cherry and satiating healthy fat will blunt your cravings and leave you feeling satisfyingly full. This shake requires no pre-soaking, making it handy for mornings on the run.

2 cups unsweetened almond milk
1 tablespoon raw cacao powder
3 ice cubes
½ cup frozen cherries (about 10 cherries)
¼ cup cooked yam, peeled*
3 dried dates, pitted
1 tablespoon coconut or MCT oil
Pinch of sea salt or pink Himalayan salt

Place the almond milk, cacao powder, ice cubes, cherries, cooked yam, dried dates, coconut oil, and salt in a high-speed blender. Blend until smooth.

To serve, pour into two glasses.

* For a quick, cooked yam, steam a whole yam in a covered pot over water on high for 10 minutes. Once it cools, peel and measure out the amount needed for the recipe. Save any remaining yam for another meal.

Detoxifier Shake

SERVES: 2

SOAK TIME: 6 hours or overnight

PREP TIME: 5 minutes

COOK TIME: 35 minutes (using a pressure cooker or multi-cooker)

Mung (or moong) beans are tridoshic, meaning they are balancing to all three doshas. Mung beans are a powerful tool for detoxing and also support an increased metabolism. This mild, warm drink is like a soup. Make sure to drink lots of water throughout the day afterward.

½ cup green mung beans
4 cups filtered water, plus more for soaking
1 teaspoon coconut oil
½ teaspoon cumin seeds
¼ teaspoon fennel seeds
¼ teaspoon turmeric powder
¼ teaspoon coriander powder
¼ teaspoon black salt or dulse
2 tablespoons lime juice

In a medium-size bowl, presoak the mung beans in enough water (about 2 cups) to cover and allow room for expansion. Soak for a minimum of 6 hours or overnight. Drain and set aside.

On the stove top: Place a medium-size pot over medium heat and add the coconut oil. When it has heated, add the cumin, fennel, turmeric, and coriander. Allow to cook for 1 minute or until fragrant. Add the soaked mung beans and 4 cups of filtered water. Bring to a boil, then lower the temperature, cover the pot, and simmer until cooked, approximately 2 hours.

In a multi-cooker: Set the pot to Sauté. Add the coconut oil and heat. Add the cumin, fennel, turmeric, and coriander. Allow to cook for 1 minute or until fragrant. Add soaked mung beans and 4 cups of filtered water. Press Cancel. Cover the pot with the lid, press the Bean button (or set it for 30 minutes). The unit will ding when ready.

Uncover the pot, pour the entire pot of beans and liquid into an appropriate-size high-speed blender. Add the black salt and 1 tablespoon lime juice and secure the lid. As a precaution, place a folded towel over the blender lid before turning on the unit. Hot liquids have a tendency to spit up to the lid and could burn your hand. With the towel in place, blend until the mixture forms a smooth soup. Taste and add more lime juice if you want a brighter flavor.

To serve, pour into two mugs.

Salud Shake

SERVES: 2
SOAK TIME: 10 minutes
PREP TIME: 10 minutes

This shake maximizes the nutritional power of green vegetables with omega-3 fatty acids in the form of flax meal. Think of it as a liquid salad with a really healthy dressing. Start your day with this shake and you'll feel energized and clear headed.

1 tablespoon flax meal or flax oil
5 ounces coconut water
1 cup packed spinach
1 small head of romaine lettuce, about 2 cups
3-inch piece peeled cucumber
¼ cup packed parsley leaves, thick stems removed
½ avocado, peel removed
2 tablespoons lime juice
7 ounces filtered water
1 small red apple, peeled and cored
1 micro-spoon powdered stevia or 2 drops liquid stevia
Pinch of salt
3 cubes ice (optional)

Presoak the flax meal (if using) in a small bowl with the coconut water. Allow to soak for 10 minutes or until soft. Do not drain. Set aside until ready to use.

In a small pot over high heat, steam the spinach in water until soft about 1 minute. Drain and set aside to cool.

Meanwhile, prep the lettuce, cucumber, parsley, avocado, and apple.

Add the cooked spinach and soaked flax meal in the coconut water (or the flax oil and coconut water), cucumber, lettuce, parsley, avocado, lime juice, water, apple, stevia, and salt to a high-speed blender. Blend until smooth, adding additional water if you prefer a more liquid shake or the ice cubes if you prefer a colder shake.

To serve, pour into two glasses.

Pitta Meals and Snacks

Several of the pitta recipes require you soak seeds, nuts, or legumes for at least 6 hours or overnight. Get in the habit of soaking them the night before you make a recipe. Most meal recipes are for two meal portions, but if you are having one as a snack (or light meal) instead, you will have four snack portions. Each recipe provides the number of portions for both a meal and a snack. Unless you are doing CLEAN7 with a partner, have one meal portion and refrigerate the other half for the following day. Some meals require a pitta-acceptable vegetable side dish to complete the meal. If you make a recipe as a snack, you will usually have three snack portions to refrigerate or freeze for another time. Most people with a pitta dosha should eat lime rather than lemon. If you get tired of lime, a good alternative is the spice sumac, which has a natural citrus flavor.

Chickpea Street Tacos

SERVES: 2 (2 TACOS) AS A MEAL
SERVES: 4 (1 TACO) AS A SNACK
PREP TIME: 10 minutes (active)
COOK TIME: 20 minutes

You won't miss the corn with these delicious tacos. The chickpea pancake folds like a soft taco. Chimichurri, a flavorful Latin herb sauce, replaces salsa. You might find you like it so much that you'll want to put it on everything!

½ cup chickpea (garbanzo bean) flour
½ cup filtered water
¼ teaspoon sea salt or pink Himalayan salt
¼ teaspoon baking soda
1 teaspoon minced green onion (green part only)
1 tablespoon avocado oil, divided
1 (6- to 8-ounce) chicken breast, diced*
1 white or brown mushroom, thinly sliced
¼ cup chopped zucchini
¼ cup chopped yellow squash
½ cup tightly packed spinach
1 avocado, peeled and sliced
1 teaspoon nutritional yeast flakes (optional)

FOR THE CHIMICHURRI SAUCE
1 green onion, roughly chopped
½ cup Italian parsley, thick stems removed
¼ cup cilantro, thick stems removed
1 shallot (about the size of a tablespoon),
    peeled and roughly chopped
¼ cup lime juice
¼ cup extra-virgin olive oil
¼ teaspoon sea salt or pink Himalayan salt (or to taste)

In a medium-size bowl, whisk the chickpea flour, filtered water, salt, baking soda, and 1 teaspoon of the green onion until smooth. Set aside.

In a large skillet over medium heat, heat 2 teaspoons of avocado oil. Add the chicken and allow it to brown, about 3 minutes, turning midway. Add the mushrooms, zucchini, yellow squash, and spinach. Cook 2 more minutes, making sure the chicken is fully cooked. Remove the skillet from the burner, cover, and set aside.

Place the remaining green onion, parsley, cilantro, shallot, and lime juice in the bowl of a food processor and pulse until well minced. Drizzle the olive oil through the chute while the processor is running until well incorporated. Using a flexible spatula, scrape the mixture into a small bowl. Mix in the salt and set aside.

Place a large cast-iron pan over medium heat on the cooktop. Add 1 teaspoon of avocado oil. Once a drop of water sizzles in the pan, scoop ¼ cup of the chickpea batter into the pan, spreading the mix until it is the size of a small tortilla. Cook until you see little bubbles forming on the top, about 30 to 40 seconds, then, using a thin spatula, flip the "tortilla" and cook for another 30 to 40 seconds. Remove from the skillet and place on a plate. Repeat three more times.

To serve, place two tortillas on each plate for a meal (or one for a snack). Distribute the avocado slices evenly over the tortillas. Top with equal portions of the chicken and vegetable mixture. For a snack, omit the vegetable mixture. Drizzle ½ teaspoon of the chimichurri sauce over each taco and sprinkle with a pinch of optional nutritional yeast.

Refrigerate leftover chicken and vegetables in a container with a lid. Place a piece of parchment paper between each leftover tortilla, place in a separate lidded container, and refrigerate.

* Use only free-range or pasture-raised chicken.

Kitchari

SERVES: 2 AS A MEAL
SERVES: 4 AS A SNACK
SOAK TIME: 6 hours or overnight
PREP TIME: 7 minutes
COOK TIME: 30 minutes (in a multi-cooker)

The ultimate Ayurvedic detox meal, this dish is tridoshic, means it is suitable for all three doshas. Yellow mung (or moong) dal is a delicate legume that cooks quickly and is easy to digest. If you can't find it at your local store, it is readily available on online.

¼ cup yellow mung dal
¼ cup basmati rice
2 cups filtered water, plus more for soaking
2 tablespoons coconut oil
1 small onion
1 small zucchini
1 small carrot
½ teaspoon cumin seeds
¼ teaspoon ground turmeric
¼ teaspoon fennel seeds
¼ teaspoon ground coriander
½ teaspoon sea salt or pink Himalayan salt
1 tablespoon lime juice
Cilantro, for garnish (optional)

In a medium-size bowl, combine the mung dal and basmati rice with enough filtered water to cover. Allow to soak for a minimum of 6 hours or overnight. Strain in a mesh strainer and set aside.

Add the onion, zucchini, and carrot to a food processor. Pulse until finely chopped.

On the stove top: Place a small pot over medium heat. Add the coconut oil and heat. Add the mix of onion, zucchini, and carrot along with the cumin, turmeric, fennel, and coriander. Allow to cook for

1 to 2 minutes. Then add the dal and rice mixture and 2 cups of filtered water. Bring to a boil, then lower the temperature, cover the pot, and simmer until cooked, approximately 2 hours.

In a multi-cooker: Set pot to Sauté. Add the coconut oil and allow it to heat. Add the vegetable mix, cumin, fennel, turmeric, and coriander. Allow to cook for 1 to 2 minutes. Add the dal and rice mixture and 2 cups of water. Press Cancel. Cover the pot with the lid, press the Bean button (or set it for 30 minutes). The pot will ding when the meal is ready.

Once cooked, uncover the pot, add salt and lime juice, and gently mix until evenly incorporated.

To serve as a meal, divide the mixture evenly between two bowls and sprinkle with optional minced cilantro.

To serve as a snack, pour one-quarter of the mixture into a small bowl and sprinkle with optional cilantro.

Waffle Hash Open-Face Sandwich

SERVES: 2 (2 TOASTS) AS A MEAL

SERVES: 4 (1 TOAST) AS A SNACK

SOAK TIME: 10 minutes

PREP TIME: 10 minutes

COOK TIME: 10 minutes

A healthier version of avocado toast, this recipe is easiest to make with a waffle iron, but if you don't have one, just make them as you would a pancake. The flax meal provides the binding you would normally get from an egg.

1 tablespoon flax meal

2 tablespoons warm filtered water

1 sweet potato, grated or noodled (using a spiralizer)

1 small onion, peeled and sliced

3 tablespoons white rice flour

1 tablespoon arrowroot

½ teaspoon sea salt or pink Himalayan salt

1 tablespoon coconut oil, melted

Avocado or sunflower oil cooking spray

8 asparagus spears, sliced in half lengthwise

2 red radishes, thinly sliced

1 avocado, peeled and mashed with a squeeze of lime
   and pinch of salt

4 slices (2 ounces each) cooked turkey or chicken breast*

Ground black pepper, to taste

1 scallion, minced (optional)

In a small cup or bowl, combine the flax meal with 2 tablespoons of warm filtered water. Set aside to soak for about 5 minutes.

Place the sweet potato and onion in a large bowl with white rice flour, arrowroot, salt, and melted coconut oil. Mix until well combined. Add the presoaked flax meal and mix well.

Turn the waffle iron to the highest setting per the instruction manual. Once ready, mist the waffle iron with avocado or sunflower oil. Add ⅓ cup of the sweet potato mix to the waffle iron, carefully spreading the mixture so that a thin layer fills the waffle cavity. Close the lid and cook for 5 minutes. The waffle iron may indicate it's ready before then but allow the sweet potato mixture to cook as close to 5 minutes as possible without burning. Once crisp, set the waffle aside on a cooling rack. Repeat until all the batter is used. Set the waffles aside on a cooking rack and keep them warm in a low oven.

Discard the fibrous ends of the asparagus and cut the spears so they are the length of the waffles. Place the asparagus and radishes in a small pot of boiling water. Allow to cook for 1 to 2 minutes, or until the vegetables are soft but not mushy. Drain and set aside.

To serve as a meal, spread equal amounts of the mashed avocado over the four hash toasts. Layer on equal amounts of asparagus and radish. Roll each slice of chicken (or turkey) and cut in half. Place two pieces of rolled chicken on top of each toast. Garnish with a dash of black pepper and a pinch of minced scallion.

As a snack, serve as above but with just 1 waffle toast.

* Use free-range or pasture-raised turkey or chicken.

Tur-Veggie Patty

SERVES: 4 (1 PATTY) AS A MEAL
SERVES: 8 (1 SMALL PATTY) AS A SNACK
PREP TIME: 10 minutes
COOK TIME: 10 minutes

My favorite way to eat a ground patty is with loads of veggies mixed in. Besides tasting great, this is also a fantastic way to get more vegetables into your diet. This tur-veggie mix can be stored in a refrigerator for up to five days or in the freezer for two weeks, making it particularly handy for times when you have little time to prepare a meal.

¼ cup hulled sunflower seeds
2 cups filtered water for soaking
2 peeled shallots, divided
1 small zucchini, roughly chopped
¼ cup parsley, thick stems removed
1 carrot, roughly chopped
2 kale leaves, stems removed or 1 packed cup of spinach
10 cremini or white mushrooms, divided
½ teaspoon dried tarragon (optional)
½ teaspoon granulated garlic
¼ teaspoon ground cumin
½ teaspoon dried basil
½ teaspoon sea salt or pink Himalayan salt
1 pound ground white turkey (or chicken) meat*
2 tablespoons avocado oil, divided
4 green lettuce leaves
1 avocado, pit removed, sliced

LIME VINAIGRETTE
¼ cup lime juice
1 teaspoon flax oil
1 tablespoon nutritional yeast flakes
¼ teaspoon sea salt or pink Himalayan salt

¼ teaspoon ground black pepper
¼ teaspoon granulated garlic
1 micro-spoon powdered stevia or 1 drop liquid stevia
½ cup extra-virgin olive oil

Place the sunflower seeds in a large bowl with 2 cups of water to soak for 6 hours minimum or overnight. Strain, rinse, and set aside.

Place the soaked seeds, 1 shallot, zucchini, parsley, carrot, kale (or spinach), 4 mushrooms, tarragon, granulated garlic, cumin, basil, and salt in a food processor, and pulse until well minced.

In a large bowl, mix the turkey with the minced vegetables until well incorporated. Shape into four same-size patties and place on a baking sheet. For snack portions, form eight smaller same-size patties.

In a large frying pan over medium heat, add 1 tablespoon of avocado oil. Once warm, place the patties in the pan and cook until brown, about 3 minutes. Flip and repeat for other side, about 3 minutes or until fully cooked.

While the patties are cooking, slice the remaining 6 mushrooms and thinly slice the remaining shallot. In a smaller frying pan, add a tablespoon of avocado oil and the sliced mushrooms and shallot. Cook until lightly browned on both sides. Set aside.

For the dressing: Place the lime juice, flax oil, nutritional yeast flakes, salt, black pepper, granulated garlic, stevia, and extra-virgin olive oil in a mason jar. Tighten the lid and shake vigorously until well mixed.

To serve as a meal, add a dollop of dressing to each lettuce leaf and top with a meal-size patty. Evenly distribute the sliced avocado and top with the cooked mushrooms and shallots.

For a snack, serve as above, but cut each lettuce leaf in half and top with a snack-size patty.

* Use free-range or pasture-raised turkey or chicken.

Bella Bites

SERVES: 2 AS A MEAL

SERVES: 4 AS A SNACK

PREP TIME: 5 minutes

COOK TIME: 15 minutes

This dish is inspired by the Shake 'n Bake style of cooking that was so popular in the 1970s. This gluten-free version uses seeds instead of bread crumbs to give the chicken a crisp texture. Don't limit this dish to just chicken. You can use fish as well! These bites are so packed with flavor they need no sauce.

Avocado oil spray, for pan

½ cup raw pepitas (pumpkin seeds)

¼ teaspoon dried mint

¼ teaspoon ground coriander

¼ teaspoon ground black pepper

½ teaspoon fennel seed

½ teaspoon cumin seed

½ teaspoon dried parsley

½ teaspoon granulated onion

½ teaspoon sea salt or pink Himalayan salt

1 tablespoon nutritional yeast

8 ounces chicken tenders, chicken breast,
   or fillets of freshwater fish*

1 tablespoon extra-virgin olive oil

Preheat the oven to 400°F. Lightly mist a baking sheet with avocado oil.

Make the crust: Place the raw pepitas, dried mint, ground coriander, black pepper, fennel seed, cumin seed, dried parsley, granulated onion, salt, and nutritional yeast in the bowl of a food processor, and process until very fine. Empty into a medium-size bowl.

Cut the chicken tenders, chicken breast, or fish fillets into bite-size pieces. Place in a small bowl with the olive oil. Toss to mix.

Dredge a couple of pieces of chicken or fish in the crust mix until both sides are well coated. Place on the greased baking sheet and repeat with the other pieces. Place the baking sheet in the oven and cook for 5 to 7 minutes. Flip over, using a thin spatula, and cook another 5 to 7 minutes or until the chicken or fish is fully cooked. Its thickness will determine the cooking time.

Remove from the oven and cool for about two to three minutes before serving.

If serving as a meal, accompany with a side dish of pitta-appropriate vegetables.

* Use free-range or pasture-raised chicken or sustainable wild-caught fish.

Quinoa Tabouleh

SERVES: 2 AS A MAIN DISH

SERVES: 4 AS A SNACK

SOAK TIME: 1 hour or overnight

PREP TIME: 5 minutes

COOK TIME: 20 minutes

Quinoa (pronounced keen-wah) is an ancient grain originally from South America. High in protein and with a nutty taste, it is a great gluten-free substitute for bulgur wheat in this refreshing and filling Lebanese-inspired salad.

½ cup uncooked quinoa

¾ cup filtered water plus more for soaking

1 carrot, roughly chopped

1 red radish

1 shallot clove, roughly chopped

1 bunch Italian parsley, thick stems removed (about 1 cup)

8 fresh mint leaves

2 tablespoons lime juice

4 tablespoons extra-virgin olive oil

½ cup diced cucumber

½ cup diced jicama (optional)

½ teaspoon sea salt or pink Himalayan salt

½ teaspoon sumac (optional)

In a medium-size bowl, combine the quinoa with enough filtered water to cover. Allow to soak for minimum of 1 hour or overnight. Use a fine mesh strainer to drain the water. Set the quinoa aside.

Place the quinoa in a large dry skillet over medium heat to dry it. Watch the pan closely, stirring the quinoa with a wooden spatula so it doesn't burn, for about 5 minutes.

Put ¾ cup of filtered water in a medium-size pot and bring to a boil. Add the quinoa, cover, and return to a boil. Turn off the heat and cover the pot for minimum of 15 minutes or until all the water has been absorbed.

While the quinoa is cooking, place the carrot, radish, shallot, parsley, and mint leaves in the bowl of a food processor. Pulse until minced but not mushy.

Empty the still warm quinoa into a large bowl, with the minced vegetables, cucumber, jicama, extra-virgin olive oil, lemon juice, salt, and sumac. Mix until well incorporated.

For a meal, place two equal portions on plates or save one for another meal. Accompany with a pitta dosha–appropriate vegetable side dish.

For a snack, place one-quarter of the tabouleh on a plate and refrigerate the rest.

NOTE: While tabouleh is traditionally eaten cold, adding the vegetables to the warm quinoa allows them to slightly steam with the still warm quinoa before eating, which is important for those with a pitta dosha. Thereafter, the dish can be eaten cold if desired.

Fakora

SERVES: 2 OR 3 (6 OR 7 PATTIES) AS A MEAL
SERVES: 5 (4 PATTIES) AS A SNACK
PREP TIME: 5 minutes
COOK TIME: 25 minutes

This recipe was inspired by Egyptian and Levantine falafel and the Indian pakora, both of which are usually deep fried. This healthier version is baked instead. It is made with lots of veggies and just a little chickpea flour. Eat the patties dry, or pair them with pesto or chimichurri sauce (page 231).

Avocado oil spray, for pan
2 tablespoons extra-virgin olive oil
1 sweet potato, roughly chopped
½ cauliflower head, roughly chopped
1 medium onion, thinly sliced
1 teaspoon grated fresh ginger
1 cup chopped spinach
¼ cup chopped cilantro
½ teaspoon ground turmeric
½ teaspoon cumin seed
1 teaspoon sea salt or pink Himalayan salt
½ teaspoon sumac
1½ cups chickpea (garbanzo bean) flour
¼ to ½ cup filtered water

Preheat oven to 425°F. Lightly spray a baking sheet with avocado oil.

Place 2 tablespoons of olive oil, the sweet potato, cauliflower, onion, fresh ginger, spinach, cilantro, ground turmeric, cumin seed, salt, sumac, and chickpea flour in the bowl of a food processor. Pulse until well mixed, but still slightly chunky. If the mix looks too dry, add ¼ cup of water and pulse again. If still too dry, add another ¼ cup water and pulse.

Using a tablespoon, scoop out 20 portions, form into patties, and place on the greased baking sheet.

Bake for 10 minutes, then use a spatula to flip over the patties. Spray with avocado oil or brush each piece with more olive oil and bake another 15 minutes, until golden brown.

Let cool on the sheet tray for 5 minutes before eating. Store the leftover patties in a container with a lid in the refrigerator for up to two weeks or in the freezer for up to two months.

If serving as a meal, accompany with a pitta dosha–appropriate vegetable as a side dish.

Kapha Recipes

Shakes

People with a Kapha constitution should avoid cold foods and drinks. Use room temperature filtered water, plant milks, and coconut water. Allow your shake to reach room temperature prior to drinking. If you use frozen berries or other fruit, also let them come to room temperature. Some of the shake recipes heat certain ingredients for this reason.

All shake recipes are for two portions. Unless you are doing CLEAN7 with a partner, refrigerate one portion and have the other half in the evening or late afternoon. Or halve a recipe if you want to try a different shake for dinner.

Most of the following shake recipes require you presoak nuts or legumes for at least 6 hours and up to 24 hours. Get in the habit of soaking them the night before you plan to make a certain shake. However, the Black Forest Shake requires no soaking and the Island Strong and Salud Shakes need just 10 minutes of soaking.

If you forget to soak ingredients, the Island Strong and Black Forest shakes don't require any presoaking and the Salud Shake only needs 10 minutes of soaking.

Island Strong Shake

SERVES: 2
PREP TIME: 5 minutes
COOK TIME: 2 minutes

Inspired by the mango lassi drink traditionally served at Indian restaurants, my dairy-free twist is to use rice milk. Lime juice and lime zest help the flavor pop. This shake substitutes papaya, another island fruit, for mango, which those with a kapha dosha should avoid. In lieu of rice milk, substitute ¼ cup of cooked basmati rice and 14 ounces of water. If you use frozen papaya, let the shake come to room temperature before drinking it.

2 cups unsweetened, unflavored rice milk
4 dried unsulfured apricots
¾ cup fresh or frozen papaya
1 tablespoon chia seeds
½ teaspoon lime juice
Pinch of lime zest
½ teaspoon fresh grated ginger
1 micro-spoon powdered stevia or 2 drops liquid stevia

Soak the chia seeds in a bowl with the rice milk for 10 minutes or until the seeds are soft.

Heat the rice milk with chia seeds and dried apricots, plus the papaya (only if frozen) in a small sauce pot for about 2 minutes until warm, but do not bring it to a boil.

Place the warm rice milk, chia seeds, apricots, and papaya, plus the lime juice, lime zest, grated ginger, and stevia in a high-speed blender. Blend until smooth.

Divide into two glasses and serve at room temperature.

Soother Shake

SERVES: 2

SOAK TIME: 6 hours or overnight

PREP TIME: 5 minutes

COOK TIME: 2 minutes

Sunflowers induce happiness. Maybe that's why I love mixing sunflower seeds in shakes. Soaking the seeds makes them both more nutritious and more smooth. Blanched almonds are okay for kapha dosha if eaten in extreme moderation. For this reason, rice milk is an option or substitute a ½ cup of cooked basmati rice with 14 ounces of filtered water.

½ cup hulled sunflower seeds

2 cups filtered water

1 tablespoon chia seeds

2 cups unsweetened, unflavored almond milk or rice milk

2 tablespoons canned 100 percent pumpkin puree
   (not pumpkin pie mix)

¼ teaspoon cinnamon

¼ teaspoon cardamom powder (optional)

½ teaspoon alcohol-free vanilla extract or vanilla powder
   (ground vanilla bean)

1 micro-spoon powdered stevia or 2 drops liquid stevia

½ cup pomegranate juice (100 percent juice,
   not from concentrate)

In a medium-size bowl, presoak the sunflower seeds in enough water to cover with room for expansion (about 2 cups water). Soak for at least 6 hours or overnight.

Drain and set the seeds aside.

Presoak the chia seeds in a small pot with the almond milk for 10 minutes or until soft. Do not drain.

Transfer the almond milk and chia seeds mixture to the stove top and cook over medium heat for about 2 minutes until warm, but not boiling.

Pour into a high-speed blender and add the drained sunflower seeds, pumpkin puree, cinnamon, optional cardamom powder, vanilla extract, stevia, and pomegranate juice. Blend until smooth.

Divide into two glasses and serve at room temperature.

Tiger's Milk Shake

SERVES: 2

SOAK TIME: 24 hours

PREP TIME: 5 minutes

This is my take on horchata, a Latin grain-based drink also known as the Gods' Nectar. Tiger nuts aren't actually nuts, but tubers with a sweet taste reminiscent of coconut. Tiger nuts require a longer soak time than nuts, seeds, or legumes do. If you can't find them, substitute sunflower seed butter.

¼ cup tiger nuts (peeled, ideally) or 1 tablespoon unsweetened
   sunflower seed butter

2¾ cups water, divided

1 tablespoon chia seeds

1 cup unsweetened, unflavored rice milk

¼ cup cooked basmati rice

3 dates, pitted, or 1 micro-spoon powdered stevia
   or 2 drops liquid stevia

½ teaspoon cinnamon

½ teaspoon alcohol-free vanilla extract or vanilla powder
   (ground vanilla bean)

Pinch of sea or pink Himalayan salt

Pinch of cardamom powder (optional)

Pinch of ginger powder (optional)

Pinch or turmeric powder (optional)

In a medium-size bowl, soak the tiger nuts in 2 cups of water for a minimum of 24 hours. Drain and set aside.

Place the chia seeds in a small bowl with the rice milk. Allow to soak for 10 minutes or until the seeds are soft. Set aside without draining.

Add the soaked chia seeds and rice milk, soaked tiger nuts, basmati rice, dates, ¾ cup of water, cinnamon, vanilla extract and salt to a high-speed blender. Blend until smooth.

Pour into two glasses and serve at room temperature. Sprinkle with a pinch each of optional cardamom, ginger, and turmeric, if desired.

Berry Blast Shake

SERVES: 2

SOAK TIME: 6 hours

PREP TIME: 5 minutes

Berries are flavorful without being too sweet—or at least as sweet as many other fruits. The only berry that is off limits during the cleanse is strawberry. Otherwise, choose the mix of berries you most enjoy.

¼ cup hulled sunflower seeds

1½ cups filtered water

1 tablespoon chia seeds

1¼ cups unsweetened rice milk

1 cup mixed fresh or frozen berries (raspberry, blueberry, and blackberry)

½ cup raw spinach

1 tablespoon lemon juice

½ teaspoon fresh grated ginger

1 micro-spoon powdered stevia or 2 drops liquid stevia

Soak the sunflower seeds in the filtered water for 6 hours or overnight. Drain and set aside the sunflower seeds.

Soak the chia seeds in a bowl with the rice milk for 10 minutes or until the seeds are soft. Do not drain. Set aside.

Add the rice milk and chia seeds, along with the soaked sunflower seeds, berries, spinach, lemon juice, grated ginger, and stevia to a high-speed blender. Blend until smooth.

Divide into two glasses and serve. If you used frozen berries, allow to come to room temperature.

Black Forest Shake

SERVES: 2
PREP TIME: 5 minutes
COOK TIME: 1 minute

When you need a chocolate fix, reach for this shake. Because it is processed, high-sugar chocolate is not supported in Ayurveda, but raw cacao powder is. A hint of cherry and some healthy fat will satiate your cravings and leave you feeling full. You can always substitute a ½ cup of cooked basmati rice and 14 ounces of water for the rice milk. This shake requires no presoaking, making it handy for mornings on the run.

2 cups unsweetened, unflavored rice milk
1 tablespoon raw cacao powder
½ cup frozen cherries (about 10 cherries)
¼ cup canned 100 percent pumpkin puree (not pumpkin pie mix) or
   canned butternut squash
1 micro-spoon powdered stevia or 2 drops liquid stevia

Heat the rice milk in a small pot with the frozen cherries on the stove top until warm, but not boiling, about 2 minutes.

Add the warm rice milk with cherries, cacao powder, pumpkin puree, and stevia to a high-speed blender and blend until smooth.

Pour into two glasses and serve.

Detoxifier Shake

SERVES: 2
SOAK TIME: 6 hours or overnight
PREP TIME: 5 minutes
COOK TIME: 35 minutes (if using a pressure cooker)

Mung (or moong) beans are tridoshic, meaning they are balancing to all three doshas. Mung beans are a powerful tool for detoxing and also support an increased metabolism. This mild, warm drink is like a soup. Make sure to drink lots of water throughout the day afterward.

½ cup dried green mung beans
6 cups filtered water, divided
1 teaspoon coconut oil
½ teaspoon cumin seeds
¼ teaspoon fennel seeds
¼ teaspoon turmeric powder
¼ teaspoon coriander powder
2 tablespoons lemon juice
¼ teaspoon black salt or dulse

In a medium-size bowl, soak the mung beans in about 2 cups of filtered water (or enough to cover them with room for expansion) for at least 6 hours or overnight. Drain and set the beans aside.

On the stove top: Add the coconut oil to a medium-size pot and place over medium heat. After the oil has heated, add the cumin, fennel, turmeric, and coriander. Allow to cook for 1 minute or until fragrant. Add the soaked mung beans and 4 cups of water. Bring mix to a boil, then lower the temperature, cover the pot and simmer until cooked, approximately 2 hours.

In a multi-cooker: Set the pot to Sauté. Add the oil, allowing it to heat. Then add the cumin, fennel, turmeric and coriander. Cook for 1 minute or until fragrant. Add the soaked mung beans and 4 cups of water. Press Cancel. Cover the pot with the lid and press the Bean button (or set it for 30 minutes). The unit will ding when the beans are ready.

Uncover either pot, pour the entire pot of beans and liquid into an appropriate-size high-speed blender. Add the salt and 1 table-spoon lemon juice and secure the lid. As a precaution, place a folded towel over the blender lid before turning on the unit. Hot liquids have a tendency to spit up to the lid and could burn your hand. With the towel in place, blend until the mixture forms a smooth soup. Taste and add more lemon juice if you want a brighter flavor.

To serve, pour into two mugs.

Salud Shake

SERVES: 2

SOAK TIME: 10 minutes

PREP TIME: 10 minutes

This shake maximizes the nutrient density of green vegetables with omega-3 fatty acids in the form of chia seeds. Think of it as a liquid salad with a really healthy dressing. A great way to start your day, it will leave you feeling energized and clearheaded.

1 tablespoon chia seeds

5 ounces coconut water

7 ounces filtered water

½ cup cauliflower florets and stems

3-inch piece peeled cucumber

1 small romaine lettuce head, about 2 cups

½ cup packed spinach

¼ cup packed parsley leaves, thick stems removed

2 tablespoons lime juice

1 small green apple, peeled and cored

1 micro-spoon powdered stevia or 2 drops liquid stevia

Pinch of sea salt or pink Himalayan salt

Soak the chia seeds in a small bowl with the coconut water for 10 minutes or until the seeds are soft. Set aside without draining.

Meanwhile, in a small pot over high heat, steam the cauliflower over filtered water until soft (about 3 minutes). Drain and set aside to cool.

Peel the cucumber, prepare the lettuce, spinach, and parsley, and peel and core the apple.

Add the coconut water with the chia seeds, the cooked cauliflower, the cucumber, lettuce, spinach, parsley, lime juice, apple, and stevia to a high-speed blender. Blend until smooth. Add additional water if you like a more liquid shake.

Pour into two glasses and serve.

Kapha Meals and Snacks

Several of the kapha recipes require you soak seeds, nuts, or legumes for at least 6 hours or overnight. Get in the habit of soaking them the night before you prepare a dish. Most recipes are for two meal portions, but if you are having one as a snack (or light meal) instead, you will have four snack portions. Each recipe provides the number of portions for both a meal and a snack. Unless you are doing CLEAN7 with a partner, you can have one meal portion and refrigerate the other half for the following day. Some meals require a kapha dosha–appropriate vegetable side dish to complete the meal. If you make a recipe as a snack, you will usually have three snack portions to refrigerate or freeze for another time. Being kapha dominant, you'll want to limit chilled foods and drinks. Warm or room temperature meals are ideal.

Chickpea Street Tacos

SERVES: 2 (2 TACOS) AS A MEAL
SERVES: 4 (1 TACO) AS A SNACK
PREP TIME: 10 minutes (active)
COOK TIME: 20 minutes

You won't miss the corn with these delicious tacos. The chickpea pancake folds just the way a soft taco does. A flavorful Latin herb sauce called chimichurri replaces salsa. You may find you like this sauce so much that you want to put it on everything!

½ cup chickpea (garbanzo) flour
½ cup filtered water
¼ teaspoon sea salt or pink Himalayan salt
¼ teaspoon baking soda
1 teaspoon minced green onion (green part only)
1 tablespoon almond oil (divided)
6- to 8-ounce chicken breast, diced*
1 garlic clove, sliced thin
1 red radish, sliced thin
¼ cup chopped white or cremini mushrooms
¼ cup chopped zucchini
½ cup spinach
1 teaspoon nutritional yeast flakes (optional)

CHIMICHURRI SAUCE
1 green onion, roughly chopped
½ cup Italian parsley, thick stems removed
¼ cup cilantro, thick stems removed
1 shallot (about tablespoon size), peeled and roughly chopped
¼ cup lemon juice
¼ cup sunflower oil
¼ teaspoon black salt or dulse, to taste

Make the pancakes: In a medium-size bowl, whisk the chickpea flour, water, salt, baking soda, and minced green onion until smooth. Set aside.

In a large skillet, heat 2 teaspoons of almond oil over medium heat. Once hot, add the chicken and garlic. Allow to brown for a total of about 3 minutes. Add the mushrooms, zucchini, radish, and spinach, and cook 2 more minutes, making sure the chicken is fully cooked. Remove the skillet from the burner, cover, and set aside.

Make the chimichurri sauce: Add the green onion, parsley, cilantro, shallot, and lemon juice to the bowl of a food processor and pulse until well minced. Next, drizzle the sunflower oil through the food processor chute while it is running until well incorporated. Using a flexible spatula, empty the contents into an appropriate size container or bowl. Mix in the salt or dulse and set aside.

Place a large cast-iron or non-stick pan over medium heat on the stovetop. Add about a teaspoon of sunflower oil. When a drop of water sizzles when dropped in the pan, it is hot enough to make the pancakes. Using a ¼-cup measuring cup, scoop the chickpea batter into the hot pan, spreading the mix until it is the size of a small tortilla. Cook for 30 to 40 seconds until you see little bubbles forming on the top. Using a thin spatula, flip the tortilla and cook for another 30 to 40 seconds. Remove to a plate. Repeat with the rest of the batter to make 3 more tortillas.

To serve as a main dish, place 2 tortillas on each plate. Evenly distribute the chicken and vegetables over all 4 tortillas. Drizzle a ½ teaspoon of the chimichurri sauce over each taco and sprinkle with a pinch of optional nutritional yeast.

To serve as a snack, place 1 tortilla on each plate, following the directions above.

Refrigerate leftover chicken and vegetables in a container with a lid. Place a piece of parchment paper between each tortilla, put in a separate container with a lid and refrigerate.

* Use only free-range or pasture-raised chicken.

Kitchari

SERVES: 2 AS A MEAL.

SERVES: 4 AS A SNACK

SOAK TIME: 6 hours or overnight

PREP TIME: 7 minutes

COOK TIME: 30 minutes (with a multi-cooker)

The ultimate Ayurvedic detox meal, this dish is tridoshic, meaning it is suitable for all three doshas. Yellow mung or moong dal is a delicate legume that cooks quickly and is easy to digest. If you can't find it at your local store, it is readily available on online.

¼ cup yellow mung (or moong) dal

¼ cup basmati rice

2 cups filtered water, plus more for soaking

½ small onion

1 small zucchini

1 small carrot

2 tablespoons almond oil

½ teaspoon cumin seeds

¼ teaspoon black mustard seeds

¼ teaspoon ground turmeric

¼ teaspoon ground coriander

½ teaspoon black salt or dulse

1 tablespoon lemon juice

Cilantro, for garnish (optional)

In a medium-size bowl, combine the mung dal and basmati rice with enough water to cover. Soak for minimum of 6 hours or overnight. Strain the water and set the dal aside.

Add the onion, zucchini, and carrot to the bowl of a food processor. Pulse until finely chopped.

On the stove top: Add the almond oil to a small sauce pot over medium heat. Add the chopped vegetable mix, cumin, black mustard, turmeric, and coriander. Cook for another minute or two. Add the dal and rice mixture and two cups of filtered water. Bring the mix to a boil, lower the temperature, cover the pot, and allow it to simmer until cooked—approximately 2 hours.

In a multi-cooker: Set the pot to Sauté. Add the coconut oil heat it. Add chopped vegetable mix, cumin, black mustard, turmeric, and coriander. Allow to cook for 1 to 2 minutes. Add the dal and rice mixture and 2 cups of filtered water. Press Cancel. Cover the pot with the lid, press the Bean button (or set it for 30 minutes). The pot will ding when the meal is ready.

Uncover the pot, add salt and lemon juice, and gently mix until evenly incorporated.

To serve as a meal, divide the meal into two bowls and sprinkle with the optional minced cilantro.

To serve as snack, pour one quarter of the meal into each small bowl and sprinkle with the optional minced cilantro.

Waffle Hash Open-Face Sandwich

SERVES: 2 (2 TOASTS) AS A MEAL

SERVES: 4 (1 TOAST) AS A SNACK

PREP TIME: 10 minutes

COOK TIME: 10 minutes

A healthier version of avocado toast, this recipe is easiest to make with a waffle iron, but if you don't have one, just make them as you would a pancake. The flax meal provides the binding that an egg normally provides. Be sure the cannellini beans contain only white kidney beans, water, and kombu seaweed. This recipe assumes a total of 4 toasts, with 2 per meal serving (and 4 per snack serving). However, since butternut squashes vary in size, you may wind up with more than 4 toasts. Set aside any additional hash toasts and keep them in a sealed container in the fridge for a week or up to a month in the freezer. Reheat in the toaster on a low setting before adding a topping.

1 tablespoon flax meal

2 tablespoons warm filtered water

1 butternut squash, peeled, seeds removed,
   and grated or noodled (using a spiralizer)

1 small onion, peeled and sliced

3 tablespoons white rice flour

1 tablespoon arrowroot

½ teaspoon dulse

1 tablespoon almond oil

Sunflower oil spray

8 asparagus spears, sliced in half lengthwise.

2 red radishes, thinly sliced

1 (15-ounce) can cooked cannellini beans

1 teaspoon lemon juice

4 slices of cooked turkey or chicken breast*
   (about 2 ounces per toast)

1 scallion, minced (optional)

Ground black pepper, to taste

In a small bowl, combine the flax meal with 2 tablespoons of warm filtered water. Soak for about 5 minutes.

Place the butternut squash and onions in a large bowl with the rice flour, arrowroot, dulse, and almond oil. Mix until well combined. Add the presoaked flax meal and mix well.

Turn the waffle iron to the highest setting per the instruction manual. Mist the iron with sunflower oil spray. Add ⅓ cup of the sweet potato mix to the waffle maker. Carefully spread the mixture so there is a thin layer filling the waffle cavity. Close the lid and allow to cook for 5 minutes. The waffle iron may say it is ready, but allow the sweet potato mix to cook as long as possible without burning. Once crisp, remove and set it on a cooling rack. Repeat until all the batter is used.

Discard the fibrous ends of the asparagus. Cut the spears to match the length of the waffle hash. Steam the asparagus and radishes over boiling water for 1 to 2 minutes until they are soft but not mushy. Remove and set the vegetables aside.

Drain and rinse the beans. Place in a small bowl with the lemon juice and mash with a fork.

To serve as a meal, spread the mashed beans over the four hash toasts. Add equal layers of the asparagus and radish to each toast. Roll the turkey slices and cut in half. Place two pieces on top of each toast. Add a dash of black pepper to each toast and garnish with an optional pinch of minced scallion.

As snack, prepare as above but have only 1 hash toast.

* Use free-range or pasture-raised chicken or turkey.

Tur-Veggie Patty

SERVES: 4 (1 PATTY) AS A MEAL

SERVES: 8 (1 SMALL PATTY) AS A SNACK

SOAKING TIME: 6 hours or overnight

PREP TIME: 15 minutes

COOK TIME: 10 minutes

This is my favorite way to eat a ground patty—with loads of veggies mixed in. Besides tasting great, this is also a fantastic way to get more vegetables into your diet. This turkey-veggie mix can be stored in a refrigerator for up to 5 days or in the freezer for 2 weeks, making it particularly handy for when you have little time to prepare a meal.

¼ cup hulled sunflower seeds

2 cups filtered water

2 shallots, peeled, divided

1 small zucchini, roughly chopped

¼ cup parsley, thick stems removed

1 carrot, roughly chopped

2 kale leaves, stem removed or 1 packed cup of spinach

10 cremini or white mushrooms, divided

½ teaspoon dried oregano

½ teaspoon granulated garlic

¼ teaspoon ground cumin

½ teaspoon dried thyme

½ teaspoon dulse

1 pound ground white turkey or white chicken meat*

2 tablespoons almond oil

4 green leaf lettuce leaves

1 (14-ounce) can quartered artichoke hearts (in water)

LEMON VINAIGRETTE
¼ cup lemon juice
1 teaspoon flax oil
1 tablespoon nutritional yeast flakes
¼ teaspoon black salt or dulse
¼ teaspoon ground black pepper
¼ teaspoon granulated garlic
1 micro-spoon powdered stevia or 1 drop liquid stevia
½ cup sunflower oil

Place the sunflower seeds in a large bowl with 2 cups of filtered water to soak for at least 6 hours or overnight. Strain, rinse, and set aside.

Place the soaked seeds, 1 shallot, zucchini, parsley, carrot, kale (or spinach), 4 mushrooms, oregano, granulated garlic, cumin, thyme, and dulse in the bowl of a food processor. Pulse until well minced.

In a large bowl, mix the ground turkey with the vegetable mix until well incorporated. Shape into 4 same-size patties (about 5 ounces each) for a meal, or 8 same-size small patties for snacks, and place on a baking sheet.

Add 1 tablespoon of almond oil to a large frying pan over medium heat. Once warm, place the patties in the pan and cook until brown, about 3 minutes (2 minutes for smaller patties). Flip and repeat on the other side, about another 3 minutes (2 minutes for smaller patties) or until the patties are fully cooked.

While the patties are cooking, slice the remaining 6 mushrooms and thinly slice the shallot. In a smaller frying pan, add a tablespoon of almond oil, the sliced mushroom, and the shallot. Cook until browned on both sides. Remove from the heat and set aside.

Drain the quartered artichokes.

Make the lemon vinaigrette: Place the lemon juice, flax oil, nutritional yeast flakes, salt, ground black pepper, granulated garlic, stevia, and sunflower oil in a mason jar. Tighten the lid and shake vigorously until well mixed.

To assemble a meal, add a dollop of dressing to each lettuce leaf. Place a patty on top. Evenly distribute the artichokes and top with the cooked mushrooms and shallots.

To assemble a snack, do as above, but cut the lettuce leaves in half and omit the cooked mushrooms and shallots.

Refrigerate or freeze extra patties and assemble at a later date.

* Use free-range or pasture-raised turkey or chicken.

Bella Bites

SERVES: 2 AS A MEAL

SERVES: 4 AS A SNACK

PREP TIME: 5 minutes

COOK TIME: 15 minutes

This dish is inspired by the Shake 'n Bake style of cooking that was so popular in the 1970s. This gluten-free version uses seeds instead of bread crumbs to give the chicken a crisp texture. Don't limit this dish to just chicken. You can use fish as well! These bites are so packed with flavor they need no sauce.

Sunflower oil spray, for pan

½ cup raw pepitas (pumpkin seeds)

¼ teaspoon powdered sage

¼ teaspoon ground mustard

½ teaspoon dried oregano

½ teaspoon dried thyme

½ teaspoon dried parsley

½ teaspoon granulated onion

½ teaspoon granulated garlic

½ teaspoon black salt or dulse

1 tablespoon nutritional yeast

8 ounces chicken tenders, chicken breast,
   or freshwater fish fillets*

1 tablespoon almond oil

Heat the oven to 400°F. Lightly mist a baking sheet with sunflower oil spray.

Place the raw pepitas, powdered sage, ground mustard, dried oregano, dried thyme, dried parsley, granulated onion, granulated garlic, black salt, and nutritional yeast in the bowl of a food processor and process until very fine. Empty into a medium-size bowl.

Cut the chicken or freshwater fish fillets cut into bite-size pieces. Place in a small bowl with the almond oil. Toss to mix.

Dredge a couple of pieces of chicken or fish in the bowl with the crust mix until both sides are well coated. Place on the greased tray and repeat with the other pieces.

Place the baking sheet in the oven and cook for 5 to 7 minutes. Flip over, using a thin spatula, and cook another 5 to 7 minutes or until the chicken or fish is fully cooked. Its thickness will determine cooking time.

Remove from oven and cool for about 2 to 3 minutes before serving.

For a meal, accompany with a kapha-appropriate cooked vegetable.

* Use free-range or pasture-raised chicken or sustainable wild-caught fish. (See https://www.seafoodwatch.org/seafood-recommendations.)

Quinoa Tabouleh

SERVES: 2 AS A MEAL

SERVES: 4 AS A SNACK

SOAK TIME: 1 hour or overnight

PREP TIME: 5 minutes

COOK TIME: 20 minutes

Quinoa (pronounced keen-wah) is an ancient grain originally from South America. High in protein, it has a nutty taste. It's also a great gluten-free substitute for bulgur wheat in this refreshing but filling Lebanese-inspired salad.

½ cup uncooked quinoa

¾ cup filtered water plus more for soaking

1 carrot, roughly chopped

1 finger-size piece of daikon radish (optional)

1 red radish

1 scallion, roughly chopped

1 bunch parsley, thick stems removed (about 1 cup)

8 fresh mint leaves

2 tablespoons lemon juice

4 tablespoons sunflower seed oil

½ cup diced jicama

½ teaspoon black salt or dulse

½ teaspoon sumac (optional)

In a medium-size bowl, combine the quinoa with enough water to cover. Allow to soak for minimum of 1 hour or overnight. Use a fine mesh strainer to remove the water.

Place the quinoa in a large dry skillet over medium heat to dry it out. Watch the pan closely, mixing the quinoa with a wooden spatula so it doesn't burn, for about 5 minutes.

Put ¾ cup of water in a medium-size pot, cover, and bring to a boil. Add the quinoa, cover, and return to a boil. Turn off the heat and keep the pot covered for minimum 15 minutes or until all the water has been absorbed.

While the quinoa is cooking, place the carrot, optional daikon radish, red radish, scallion, parsley, and mint leaves in the bowl of a food processor. Pulse until minced but not mushy.

Empty the still warm quinoa into a large bowl, along with the minced vegetables, jicama, lemon juice, sunflower seed oil, oil, black salt, and sumac. Mix until well incorporated.

For a meal, place two equal portions on two plates or save one for another meal. Serve with a kapha dosha–appropriate vegetable side dish.

NOTE: Tabouleh is traditionally eaten cold, but it's important that people with a kapha dosha eat this recipe at room temperature or still slightly warm.

Fakora

SERVES: 2 OR 3 (6 TO 7 PATTIES) AS A MEAL
SERVES: 5 (4 PATTIES) AS A SNACK
PREP TIME: 5 minutes
COOK TIME: 25 minutes

This recipe was inspired by Egyptian and Levantine falafel and the Indian pakora, both of which are usually deep-fried. This healthier version is baked instead. It is made with lots of veggies and just a little chickpea flour. Eat the patties dry, or pair them with pesto or chimichurri sauce (page 257).

Sunflower oil spray, for pan
2 tablespoons almond oil
2 carrots, roughly chopped
½ cauliflower head, roughly chopped
1 medium yellow onion, thinly sliced
1 teaspoon grated fresh ginger
1 cup chopped spinach
¼ cup chopped cilantro
½ teaspoon ground turmeric
½ teaspoon granulated garlic
½ teaspoon cumin seed
½ teaspoon fenugreek
1 teaspoon black salt or dulse
½ teaspoon sumac
1½ cups chickpea (garbanzo) flour
¼ to ½ cup filtered water

Heat the oven to 425°F.

Mist a baking sheet with sunflower oil spray.

Place 2 tablespoons of almond oil, the carrots, cauliflower, onion, fresh ginger, spinach, cilantro, ground turmeric, granulated garlic, cumin seed, fenugreek, black salt, sumac, and chickpea flour in the bowl of a food processor. Pulse until well mixed, but still slightly chunky. If the mix looks too dry, add ¼ cup of filtered water and pulse again. If still too dry, add the other ¼ cup water and pulse again.

Using a tablespoon, scoop out 20 portions, form into patties, and place on the greased baking sheet.

Bake for 10 minutes. Use a spatula to flip over. Spray or brush each piece with more sunflower seed oil and bake another 15 minutes, until golden brown.

Let cool on the sheet tray for 5 minutes before removing.

For a meal, divide into two or three portions and serve with a kapha dosha–appropriate vegetable side dish.

For a snack, divide into four portions.

Store the leftover patties in a sealed container in the refrigerator for up to two weeks or in the freezer for up to two months.

Celebratory Meals

Whether you've cleansed for seven or twenty-one days, you have great reason to celebrate. Changing habits around food is no easy task, but you did it! To celebrate, we've supplied a full day of food, including an alcoholic drink. However, we don't want you to just toss aside everything you've learned about yourself during the last week or three. That's why every celebratory recipe is CLEAN7 approved—well, except for the alcohol in the celebratory cocktail! CLEAN7-approved recipes follow the Elimination Diet. Put on your favorite music and smile as you make these delicious and CLEAN7 recipes. It's celebration time. The new you deserves it.

Celebratory Shake

Raspberries and Cream Shake

SERVES: 2

SOAK TIME: 10 minutes

PREP TIME: 5 minutes

I can't think of a better way to celebrate your week of detoxing than with this creamy, slightly tart smoothie. Use your favorite dairy-free vanilla protein powder. If raspberries aren't your thing, feel free to use any CLEAN7-approved fruit, such as blueberries, mango, or pineapple. Use canned coconut milk, not the beverage in a carton. Avoid coconut milk with guar gum in the ingredients list.

1 tablespoon chia seeds

1 cup canned coconut milk

1 cup fresh or frozen raspberries

1 cup filtered water

1 tablespoon unsweetened cashew butter

1 teaspoon maca powder (optional)

1 tablespoon MCT oil (optional)

1 teaspoon alcohol-free vanilla extract or vanilla powder

Dairy-free protein powder
  (portion based on packaging instructions)

4 ice cubes (optional)

Soak the chia seeds in a bowl with the coconut milk for 10 minutes or until the seeds are soft. Place the soaked chia seeds with the coconut milk, raspberries, filtered water, unsweetened cashew butter, optional maca powder, optional MCT oil, vanilla extract, protein powder, and ice cubes in a high-speed blender and pulse until smooth.

Pour into two glasses and serve.

Celebratory Breakfast

Sweet Potato Hash

SERVES: 2
PREP TIME: 5 minutes
COOK TIME: 15 minutes

This hearty egg-free breakfast will keep you satisfyingly full until lunchtime.

4 to 6 leaves of chard (any type), including stalks
1 tablespoon coconut oil
1 large sweet potato, peeled and diced (about 2½ cups)
1 small yellow onion, diced (about ½ cup)
6 ounces ground turkey*
1 teaspoon sea salt or pink Himalayan salt
½ teaspoon ground cumin
½ teaspoon ground turmeric
½ teaspoon dried thyme
½ teaspoon ground mustard
1 teaspoon nutritional yeast
1 to 2 tablespoons filtered water
¼ cup chopped raw cashews
1 teaspoon lemon juice
1 tablespoon chopped fresh parsley

Chop the chard stems and place in a small bowl. Chop the chard leaves and place in another small bowl.

In a large frying pan over medium heat, add the coconut oil. As it heats up, add the sweet potato and onion. Cook for 2 minutes. Add the ground turkey, chopped chard stalks (not leaves), salt, cumin, turmeric, thyme, mustard, and nutritional yeast. Cook for 2 minutes, mixing well with a wooden spatula. Add the water and cover with a lid to help the sweet potato soften.

After about 5 minutes remove the lid, add the cashews and chard leaves. Continue to cook for another 2 to 4 minutes or until the sweet potatoes and turkey are cooked. Remove from the heat.

Toss the hash with the lemon juice and mix well. Divide on to two plates and garnish with the chopped parsley.

* Use free-range or pasture-raised turkey.

Celebratory Lunch

Greek Salad

SERVES: 2
PREP TIME: 15 minutes
COOK TIME: 8 to 12 minutes

I love a great salad. The key to eating more salad is making sure it's easy to assemble and they don't get much easier than this main dish salad. It's also a great way to make use of leftover chicken, fish, or another protein source. If you use canned garbanzo beans, be sure to rinse them well.

6 ounces raw chicken, salmon, or lamb*
1 teaspoon extra-virgin olive oil
1 head romaine lettuce, chopped
½ cucumber, peeled and diced
½ cup cooked or canned garbanzo beans (chickpeas)
½ cup pitted kalamata olives
1 carrot, rough chopped
1 celery stalk, roughly chopped
¼ cup parsley roughly chopped
1 clove garlic

LEMON VINAIGRETTE:
1 tablespoon lemon juice
3 tablespoons extra-virgin olive oil
1 teaspoon flax oil
1 teaspoon liquid coconut nectar
¼ teaspoon sea salt or pink Himalayan salt
¼ teaspoon ground black pepper
½ teaspoon sumac

Slice the chicken, fish, or lamb into bite-size pieces. Cook in a pan with the olive oil over medium heat until fully cooked. Or place on a grill and when fully cooked, slice and set aside.

Place the chopped romaine lettuce, cucumber, and garbanzo beans in a large bowl.

Place the olives, carrot, celery, parsley, and garlic in the bowl of a food processor. Pulse until well minced. Pour into the large bowl with the other ingredients.

Place the lemon juice, 3 tablespoons olive oil, flax oil, coconut nectar, sea salt, black pepper, and sumac in a mason jar. Secure the lid tightly and shake vigorously until the dressing is well mixed.

Just prior to serving, toss the dressing with the salad until lightly coated and serve.

* Fish should be wild caught, chicken free range, and lamb pastured.

Celebratory Snack

Stuffed Mushrooms

SERVES: 2
SOAK TIME: 6 hours or overnight
PREP TIME: 5 minutes
COOK TIME: 10 minutes

Stuffed mushrooms are the perfect finger food. Easy to make and packed full of flavor, this snack will help boost your daily vegetable intake.

½ cup raw cashews or almonds
2 cups filtered water
1 cup packed spinach
1 clove garlic
1 small clove shallot
½ teaspoon granulated onion
½ teaspoon sea salt or pink Himalayan salt
1 tablespoon nutritional yeast
½ zucchini
½ carrot
6 to 8 cremini mushrooms, cleaned and destemmed
   (save the stems)
Extra-virgin olive oil

Soak the cashews or almonds in 2 cups of water, or more to cover, for a minimum of 6 hours or overnight. Drain and set the nuts aside.

Preheat the oven to 425°F. Use an oven-safe frying pan or line a rimmed baking sheet with parchment paper.

Make the stuffing: Pulse the spinach, drained nuts, garlic, shallot, onion, salt, nutritional yeast, zucchini, carrot, and mushroom stems in a small food processor.

Place the mushrooms cap-side down in the pan, add a heaping tablespoon of the stuffing, drizzle with a little olive oil, and cook for 10 minutes.

Remove from the pan, allow to cool for a few minutes, and serve.

Celebratory Drink

Refreshing Mojito

SERVES: 1

PREP TIME: 5 minutes

I don't often drink alcohol but when I do, I might well have a Mojito. I love the way the mint and lime dance together in the glass. A little grated fresh ginger and lime zest boost the refresh factor. It is best sipped through a straw.

¼ teaspoon lime zest

2 tablespoons fresh lime juice

8 to 10 fresh mint leaves

⅛ teaspoon sea salt or pink Himalayan salt

1 teaspoon monk fruit sweetener or xylitol

¼ teaspoon fresh grated ginger

2 ounces white rum

4 to 5 ice cubes

Sparkling mineral water

Lime wedges and mint sprigs for garnish

You'll want a tall, 12- to 14-ounce glass and a muddler to mix this drink. A long wooden pestle can do the job if you don't have a muddler.

Zest the lime before juicing and set the zest aside.

Add the lime juice, mint leaves, salt, monk fruit sweetener, and ginger to the glass. Using a pestle or muddler, gently press the mint leaves making sure not to tear the leaves. Overdoing it can make the drink bitter.

Pour in the rum. Add the ice cubes, then top off with 4 or more ounces of sparkling mineral water. Sprinkle on the lime zest and garnish with a lime wedge and a sprig of mint. Enjoy!

Celebratory Dinner

Sweet Mustard Salmon

SERVES: 2
PREP TIME: 5 minutes
COOK TIME: 7 minutes

I pair this easy and delicious recipe with roasted asparagus but feel free pick your favorite vegetable accompaniment.

SWEET MUSTARD SAUCE
1 clove shallot
1 clove garlic
1 teaspoon dried rosemary
1 teaspoon dried thyme
2 tablespoons liquid coconut nectar (not granulated nectar)
2 tablespoons tamari or coconut aminos
1 tablespoon lemon juice
2 tablespoons extra-virgin olive oil
2 tablespoons whole-grain mustard
1 (8-ounce) fillet of wild-caught salmon, cut in half
1 bunch asparagus (about 8 spears or more per person)
1 to 2 tablespoons extra-virgin olive oil
Zest of 1 lemon
Sea salt or pink Himalayan salt, to taste
Ground black pepper, to taste
Zested lemon

Make the sweet mustard sauce: In a small food processor, combine the shallot, garlic, rosemary, thyme, coconut nectar, tamari, lemon juice, and olive oil and blend well. Transfer to a small bowl and add the mustard. Stir to combine.

In a large bowl, toss the asparagus with the lemon zest, 1 to 2 tablespoons of extra-virgin olive oil, sea salt, and black pepper.

Preheat the broiler. Line a baking sheet with foil. Arrange the asparagus on half the baking sheet. Arrange the salmon skin side down on the other side of the sheet. Spoon the maple mustard sauce over the salmon. Broil for 5 to 7 minutes or until the salmon is cooked.

Divide the asparagus and salmon on two plates.

Celebratory Dessert

Ooey-Gooey Brownies

SERVES: 9 (2-INCH) SQUARES
SOAK TIME: 10 minutes
PREP TIME: 5 minutes
COOK TIME: 25 minutes

Nothing says celebrate like chocolate. These grain-free, eggless chocolate brownies are just the ticket to say, "Job well done!"

2 tablespoons flax meal
6 tablespoons filtered water
1 cup almond butter
⅓ cup monk fruit sweetener
2 tablespoons coconut oil
1 teaspoon alcohol-free vanilla extract or vanilla powder
   (ground vanilla bean)
⅓ cup cacao powder
½ teaspoon baking soda

Heat the oven to 350°F. Line an 8-inch square pan with parchment paper for easy removal when baked. There is no need to grease the pan.

In a small dish, add the flax meal and filtered water. Soak for 10 minutes.

In a large bowl, mix together the flax meal mixture, almond butter, monk fruit sweetener, coconut oil, vanilla, cacao, and baking soda. Pour into the prepared pan. Bake for 25 minutes or until a toothpick inserted into the center comes out clean.

Allow the brownies to cool in the pan before cutting into 9 squares.

Acknowledgments

Thank you to my immediate family for the beautiful life we share, Grace Junger, Beilo Junger, Seraphina Junger, Griffin, Lara, Pablo, Zack, and Scales. Andrea, Clementina and Manuel, Anabella and Javier.

A special thank you to Tierney Gearon for Grace, for being an awesome mom, friend, and for lifting me up when I was broken. Michael, Emilee, Walker, thank you for taking care of me at that time as well. Thank you Carla for Beilo and Fina and for being a great mom and coparent.

Thank you Richard Baskin for your mentorship and friendship. Thank you Skip and Edie Bronson for all your love and protection.

Thank you Miguel Gil for your unconditional friendship and superhero moves as double CEO. And to Yetta for her love and grace.

Thank you Bharat and Bhavani for your vision, your generosity, your love and support.

Big thanks to Fernando Sulichin and Jose Luis Longinotti, always there, unconditionally.

Thank you Gideon Weil and the *CLEAN7* team at HarperCollins: Lisa Zuniga, Sydney Rogers, Margaret Bridges, and everyone else who contributed.

Big thanks to Olivia Bell Buehl and to Andrea Barzvi. Thanks Chef James Barry for the amazing recipes.

Thank you Christian Visdomini for your help and guidance, and to the whole team at CGA.

Thank you to my CLEAN family, Sophie, Emily, Pascalle, Brian, Graham, Ashley, and Karo.

Thank you to my ORGANIC INDIA family, William Bissell, Abhinandan Doke, Mukesh, Oded, Parasher, Dinesh, Balram, Ritesh, Saurabh, Prasdad, Pankaj, Subrata, Vikram, Vandita, Raja, Vikash, Elizabeth, Arlene, and Shikha.

Special thanks to my French family, Clovis, Celine, Fiji, Jao, and everyone at La Petite Blaque.

Thank you JP Baba for helping and protecting me and to all the special friends around you, Kylie, Ben, Guy, Damien, Ian, Debbie, John, Christian, Lal, Anton, and Valeria.

Bibliography

Chapter 1

Bland, J. S., E. Barrager, R. G. Reedy, and K. Bland. November 1, 1995. "A Medical Food-Supplemented Detoxification Program in the Management of Chronic Health Problems." *Altern Ther Health Med.* 1(5):62–71.

Goel, P., K. Goel, and S. Singh. 2012. "Role of paraoxonases in detoxification of organophosphates." *JARMS.* 4(4):320–25.

Harvard Health Letter. June 2011. "Drugs in the Water." https://www.health.harvard.edu/newsletter_article/drugs-in-the-water.

Hodges, R. E. and D. M. Minich. 2015. "Modulation of Metabolic Detoxification Pathways Using Food and Food-Derived Components: A Scientific Review with Clinical Application." *J Nutr Metab.* 2015: 760689.

Pandey, M. M. and S. Rastogi. 2013. "Indian Traditional Ayurvedic System of Medicine and Nutritional Supplementation." *Evid Based Complement Alternat Med.* 2013:376327.

Yun-Hee, Youm, Y. Nguyen Kim, and W. Grant Ryan. 2015. "The ketone metabolite b-hydroxybutyrate blocks NLRP3 inflammasome-mediated inflammatory disease." *Nature Medicine.* 21:263–69.

Chapter 2

American Academy of Asthma Allergy and Immunology. 2019. "Food Intolerance versus Food Allergy" https://www.aaaai.org/conditions-and-treatments/library/allergy-library/food-intolerance.

Barbalho, S. M., et al. January–March 2016. "Inflammatory bowel disease: Can omega-3 fatty acids really help?" *Ann Gastroenterol.* 29(1):37–43.

Canani, B., et al. June 2015. "The role of commensal microbiota in the regulation of tolerance to dietary antigens." *Current Opinion in Allergy and Clinical Immunology.* 15(3):243–49.

Catterson, J. H., et al. June 4, 2018. "Short-Term Intermittent Fasting Induces Long-Lasting Gut Health and TOR-Independent Lifespan Extension." *Curr Biol.* 28(11):1714–24.

Dwivedi, M., et al. April 2016. "Induction of regulatory T cells: A role for probiotics and prebiotics to suppress autoimmunity." *Autoimmun Rev.* 15(4): 379–92.

Farnsworth, N. R., et al. 1985. "Medicinal plants in therapy." *Bul. World Health Org.* 63(6):965–81.

Hayward, S., et al. 2014. "Effects of intermittent fasting on markers of body composition and mood state." *Journal of the International Society of Sports Nutrition.* 11(1 Suppl):25.

Hicks, K., and G. Hart. 2008. "Role for food-specific IgG-based elimination Diets." *Nutrition & Food Science.* 38(5):404–16.

Kim, J., et al. December 2013. "The effects of elimination diet on nutritional status in subjects with atopic dermatitis." *Nutr Res Pract.* 7(6):488–94.

Mu, Q., et al. May 23, 2017. "Leaky Gut as a Danger Signal for Autoimmune Diseases." *Front. Immunol.* https://doi.org/10.3389/fimmu.2017.00598.

Nishteswar, K., et al. 2018. "Role of herbal prebiotics and probiotics in intestinal health / 7th annual congress on probiotics, nutrition and microbes." *J Prob Health.*6.

Seimon, R. V., et al. December 15, 2015. "Do intermittent diets provide physiological benefits over continuous diets for weight loss? A systematic review of clinical trials." *Mol Cell Endocrinol.* 418:153–72.

Skrovanek, S., et al. November 15, 2014. "Zinc and gastrointestinal disease." *World J Gastrointest Pathophysiol.* 5(4):496–513.

Wang, B., et al. 2015. "Glutamine and intestinal barrier function." *Amino Acids.* 47:2143.

Yadav, H., et al. August 30, 2013. "Beneficial metabolic effects of a probiotic via butyrate-induced GLP-1 hormone secretion." *J Biol Chem.* 288(35): 25088–97.

Chapter 3

Dionisio, A. P., R. T. Gomes, and M. Oetterer. September/October 2009. "Ionizing radiation effects on food vitamins—A Review." *Braz Arch Biol Technol.* 52(5).

Eisenstein, M. Scientific American Custom Media. September 19, 2018. "Inactive Ingredients, Active Risks." https://www.scientificamerican.com/custom-media/inactive-ingredients-active-risks/.

Kummerow, F. A. August 2009. "The negative effects of hydrogenated trans fats and what to do about them." *Atherosclerosis* 205(2):458–65.

K. U. Integrative Medicine / The University of Kansas Medical Center. 2016. "Medical Symptoms Questionnaire (MSQ)." http://www.kumc.edu/Documents/integrativemed/Medical%20Symptoms%20Questionnaire(0).pdf.

Chapter 4

Centers for Disease Control and Prevention. CDC Newsroom. 2016 (archived). "1 in 3 adults don't get enough sleep." https://www.cdc.gov/media/releases/2016/p0215-enough-sleep.html.

Hussain, J., and M. Cohen. 2018. "Clinical Effects of Regular Dry Sauna Bathing: A Systematic Review." *Evid Based Complement Alternat Med.* 2018:1857413.

Kecskes, A. A. Pacific College of Oriental Medicine. 2019. "Neurohormonal Effects of Massage Therapy." https://www.pacificcollege.edu/news/blog/2014/11/08/neurohormonal-effects-massage-therapy-1.

National Institutes of Health, 2016. "How is the body affected by sleep deprivation?"https://www.nichd.nih.gov/health/topics/sleep/conditioninfo/sleep-deprivation.

Rapaport, M. H., P. Schettler, and C. Bresee. 2010. "A preliminary study of the effects of a single session of Swedish massage on hypothalamic-pituitary-adrenal and immune function in normal individuals." *The Journal of Alternative and Complementary Medicine.* 16(10):1–10.

Rosenthal. D. S., A. Webster, and E. Ladas. 2018. "Chapter 156—Integrative Therapies in Patients with Hematologic Diseases." *Hematology. Seventh Edition.* 2253–61.

Taheri, S., et al. 2004. "Short sleep duration is associated with reduced leptin, elevated ghrelin, and increased body mass index." *PLoS Medicine.* 1(3):210217.

Chapter 7

Abdollah, T. June 13, 2008. "The 'new shower curtain smell'? It's toxic, study says." *Los Angeles Times.* https://www.latimes.com/archives/la-xpm-2008-jun-13-me-showercurtain13-story.html.

CDC Newsroom. July 18, 2017. "New CDC Report: More than 100 million Americans have diabetes and prediabetes."https://www.cdc.gov/media/releases/2017/p0718-diabetes-report.html.

Cooly, K., et al. August 31, 2009. "Naturopathic care for anxiety: a randomized controlled trial ISRCTN78958974." *PLoS One.* 4(8):e6628.

Dayani, Siriwardene S. A., et al. January 2010. "Clinical efficacy of Ayurveda treatment regimen on Subfertility with Poly Cystic Ovarian Syndrome (PCOS)." *Ayu.* 31(1):24–7.

Environmental Working Group, *EWG's Healthy Living: Home Guide.* 2007–2019. "The air inside our homes is 2 to 5 times more polluted than the air outside."

EWG Communications Team, *Environmental Working Group News*, October 28, 2009. "Toxic Cleaner Fumes Could Contaminate California Classrooms." https://www.ewg.org/news/news-releases/2009/10/28/toxic-cleaner-fumes-could-contaminate-california-classrooms.

Kanchongkittiphon, W., et al. 2015. "Indoor Environmental Exposures of Asthma: An Update to the 2000 Review by the Institute of Medicine." *Environmental Health Perspectives.* 123:6–20

Nazarroff, W.W. and C. J. Weschler. 2004. "Cleaning Products and Air Fresheners: Exposure to Primary and Secondary Air Pollutants." *Atmospheric Environment.* 38:2841–65.

Swarup A. and K. Umadevi. 1998. "Evaluation of EveCare in the treatment of Dysmenorrhoea and Premenstrual Syndrome." *Obs & Gynae. Today* (III)6:369.

Wiboonpun, N., P. Phuwapraisirisan, and S. Tip-pyang. September 2004. "Identification of antioxidant . . . compound from Asparagus racemosus." *Phytother Res.* 18(9):771–3. https://www.ewg.org/healthyhomeguide/.

Zeng, F., et al. 2017. "Occupational exposure to pesticides and other biocides and risk of thyroid cancer." *BMJ Occupational & Environmental Medicine.* 74(7).

Index

A

acetaminophen, 19
acrylamides, 18
acupuncture, 73, 99
adaptogen, 128
AFMCP (Applying Functional Medicine in Clinical Practice) course, 25–26
after photos, 105
agni (digestive fire), 37–38, 39, 40
air purification, 180–81
alcohol, 72, 76, 105–6, 155, 167, 174, 175
Alive (Read), 23
alkaline tide, 47
alkalization of water, 182
allergies: author's experience with, 24, 134; food allergy tests, 9, 27–28
aluminum, 17
aluminum lake, 19
ama (toxic obstacles), 33, 36–37, 39–40, 79, 115
Amazon, 62
ammonia, 17
animal/fish protein: CLEAN Diet foods to enjoy, 154; Combined Elimination Diet and Kapha Dosha Food List, 172, 174; Combined Elimination Diet and Pitta Dosha Food List, 168, 170; Combined Elimination Diet and Vata Dosha Food List, 164, 166; foods to avoid, 155; Kapha Dosha Food List, 162, 163; Pitta Dosha Food List, 160, 161; pre-cleanse yourself of meats, 77; pre-cleanse yourself of shrimp, 77; Vata Dosha Food List, 158, 159
animals: fight-or-flight reaction of, 110, 111, 113; follow nature's rules, 1–2, 4, 15; plant-eating vs. meat eaters, 46; rescue of sea turtle rescue, 1; toxic exposure of cats and dogs, 18
antibiotics, 17, 18
antidepressants, 17, 18
anti-inflammatories, 17, 18
antimony carbaryl, 18
antioxidants: Ayurveda herbs providing, 44, 128; CLEAN7 recipes providing, 30
anxiety: detoxing quantum toxins of, 73; meditation for calming, 114–18
apples, as Dirty Dozen food, 66
arsenic, 18

arthritis, 132–33
ashwagandha, 44, 61, 128
asparagus (Clean Fifteen), 67
Atkins diet, 12
ATP (adenosine triphosphate), 43
avocados (Clean Fifteen), 67
Ayurveda (knowledge of life), 33
Ayurvedic herbs: antimicrobial effect
    of, 29; boosting body's repair, 30;
    CLEAN7 follow-up with periodic
    detox using, 177–78; for a detox
    program, 44–45; India's "green
    revolution" impact on, 126–27;
    medicinal and healing qualities
    of, 43–45, 126, 131–33; ORGANIC
    INDIA brand recommended for, 62,
    125–31; reinoculating intestinal
    flora, 31; where to purchase, 62.
    See also medications; nutrition
Ayurvedic Medicine: on *agni* (digestive
    fire), 37–38, 39, 40; author's study
    of, 24, 32–36; CLEAN7 based on
    principles of, 7, 8; detoxification as
    traditional practice of, 13, 20, 36;
    Functional Medicine similarities
    to, 133–34; healing power of, 126,
    131–33; principles of nutrition,
    42–43. *See also* CLEAN7 program;
    medicine
Ayurvedic medicine doctors, 177
Ayurvedic thinking: on the doshas
    (body types), 38–40; on the five
    elements and nature, 38; navigating
    your life with, 40
Azamgath (Indian village), 129–31

B
Baal Shem Tov, 32
bad dreams, 73
Barry, James, 60, 187–93

beauty, 81
before-and-after photos, 68–69, 105
Belen, Susana, 24
Bella Bites recipe: kapha body type,
    266–67; pitta body type, 239–40;
    vata body type, 214–15
benzene, 17
Berry Blast Shake recipe: kapha recipe,
    251; pitta body type, 224; vata body
    type, 199
beverages: alcohol, 72, 76, 105–6, 167;
    caffeine, 72, 76, 105–6; Combined
    Elimination Diet and Kapha Dosha
    Food List, 173, 175; Combined
    Elimination Diet and Pitta
    Dosha Food List, 171; Combined
    Elimination Diet and Vata Dosha
    Food List, 165, 167
bidoshic doshas, 60
biofeedback, 31
bipolar disorder, 108
bisphenol A (BPA), 18
Black Forest Shake recipe: kapha recipe,
    252; pitta body type, 225; vata body
    type, 200
Bland, Jeffrey, 25–26
blenders, 62, 188–89
the body: cumulative effect of toxicity
    on, 19–20; evolution and disruption
    of feasting and fasting impact on,
    46–50; healing practices aligning
    nature with, 4–5; modern lifestyle
    and stresses on, 14–19; nature's rules
    for the, 1–2, 4; *Repair* (the Five Rs)
    to repair, 30. *See also* detoxification;
    doshas system
body (planetary), 134–35
boosters. *See* CLEAN7 boosters
boredom, 73–74, 93
bovine growth hormone (rBGH), 18

bowel movements, 72
Bragg, Paul, 181
brahmi, 44, 61
breakfast: historic evolution of, 50–51; skipping, 177; Sweet Potato Hash recipe, 274–75. *See also* shake recipes
breathing (mindful), 104
broccoli (Clean Fifteen), 67
Buddha, 32
butylated hydroxyanisole (BHA), 18
butylated hydroxytoluene (BHT), 18

C
cabbage (Clean Fifteen), 67
caffeine, 72, 76, 105–6
Canessa, Dr. Roberto, 22–23
canola oil, 76
cantaloupe melons (Clean Fifteen), 67
carbon filtration, 182
carboxymethylcellulose, 19
carbs as the enemy, 12
carcinogens. *See* toxins/carcinogens
cauliflower (Clean Fifteen), 67
celebrating CLEAN7 completion, 104–6
celebratory recipes: Greek Salad, 276–77; Ooey-Gooey Brownies, 283; Raspberries and Cream Shake, 273; Refreshing Mojito, 280; Stuffed Mushrooms, 278–79; Sweet Mustard Salmon, 281–82; Sweet Potato Hash, 274–75
celery (Dirty Dozen), 66
Centers for Disease Control and Prevention (CDC) study [2016], 102–3
cherries (Dirty Dozen), 66
Chickpea Street Tacos recipe: kapha recipe, 257–58; pitta body type, 231–32; vata body type, 205–6
children and medications, 19

Chimichurri Sauce recipe: kapha recipe, 257; pitta body type, 231; vata body type, 205
Chinese medicine: detoxification as traditional practice of, 13; Golden Cabinet's integrative practice of, 24–25; herbs used in, 43
chlorine, 17
chloroform, 17
chocolate: Combined Elimination Diet and Kapha Dosha Food List to avoid, 175; Combined Elimination Diet and Pitta Dosha Food List to avoid, 171; Combined Elimination Diet and Vata Dosha Food List to avoid, 167; Kapha Dosha Food List to avoid, 163; Pitta Dosha Food List to avoid, 159; Vata Dosha Food List to avoid, 155
chocolate substitution recipes: Black Forest Shake, 200, 225, 252; Ooey-Gooey Brownies recipe, 283
CLEAN (company), 134–35
CLEAN (Junger), 26, 36, 133, 134
CLEAN7 Audit, 67–68, 74–76
CLEAN7 benefits: after finishing the CLEAN7 program, 104–6, 136–38; beauty, 81; deeper sleep, 81; energy surges, 80; equanimity, 78–79; mental clarity, 78; weight loss, 79–80
CLEAN7 boosters: acupuncture, 99, colonics and enemas, 84, 91–93; detox with mindful breathing, 104; exercise, movement, and more, 84, 94–96; having fun, 84; hot and cold plunges, 84, 88–90; massage, 84; meditation, 31, 84, 96–98; rest and sleep, 84; saunas, 77, 84, 88; skin brushing, 100; sweating, 87–88
CLEAN7 enemies: bad dreams, irritability, and mood changes, 73;

CLEAN7 enemies (*continued*)
constipation, 71–72; cravings, 70;
headaches, 72–73; hunger, 69–70;
impatience and boredom, 73–74,
93; noncompliance, 74; social
pressure, 71

CLEAN7 Planner, 145–52

CLEAN7 program: brief overview of
day-by-day, 83–87; celebrating and
reflecting after completing, 104–6,
136–38; continuing to use the,
138–40; core principles of the, 7–10,
20–21; deconstructing the CLEAN7
diet and, 142; doshas (body types)
in, 40–41; overcoming fear and
barriers to, 16–19; personalizing your
own, 141; repeat periodically, 140;
the right time to embark on, 81–82;
turning practices into habits, 106–7;
as union of modern and ancient
sciences, 7, 41–43. *See also* Ayurvedic
Medicine; detoxification; Functional
Medicine; intermittent fasting

CLEAN7 program days: CLEAN7
Planner for each of the, 145–52; Day
1, 85–87, 141, 146; Day 2, 89, 141,
147; Day 3, 92, 141, 148; Day 4, 95,
141, 149; Day 5, 97, 141, 150; Day 6,
101–2, 141, 151; Day 7, 103, 141, 152

CLEAN7 program success factors:
deciding on pre-cleanse or not,
76–77; determine your Ayurvedic
dosha, 59–61; eliminate toxic foods,
63; get your Ayurvedic herbs, 61–62;
journaling, 67–68, 105; know your
enemies, 69–74; making the decision
to start, 57; use a planner, 82;
prepare your kitchen and household,
62–63; print out seven-day protocol,
58–59; set your intention on fire,

57–58; take before-and-after photos,
68–69, 105; use whole foods, 63–65

CLEAN7 program tips: consider doing
the program with someone, 77;
double shake recipe for morning
and later, 87, 93; on eating late, 90,
92–93; line up your network, 77;
make your shake the night before,
87; try on jeans on Day 1 and then
Day 7, 87

CLEAN7 protocol: printing out copy
of, 58–59; reducing your body's toxic
load using, 65; using whole foods,
63–65

CLEAN7 questionnaires: Find Your
Dosha, 156–57; the CLEAN7 Audit,
67–68, 74–76; to reveal vikriti
(momentary dosha imbalance),
41–42, 60, 61, 142; to reveal your
prakriti (primordial dosha type),
41–42, 60

CLEAN7 recipes: celebratory meals,
272–83; designed for each dosha,
60; James Barry's introduction to
the, 187–93; for kapha body type,
245–71; for pitta body type, 220–44;
providing all necessary nutrients, 30;
for vata body type, 194–219.
See also meals

CLEAN7 recipes tips: countertop
appliances, 62, 188–91; for dry
heat, 191; find your dosha, 187–88;
importance of food quality, 192–93;
on ingredients and soaking, 188;
suit your eating style and dietary
preferences, 191–92; sustaining the
benefits of CLEAN7, 193; for wet
heat, 192

CLEAN Diet–The Complete List,
154–55

The Clean Fifteen, 64, 67

CLEAN program, 26, 36

coconut carbon filter, 182

cold and hot plunges, 84, 88–90

colonics, 72, 91–93

condiments: CLEAN Diet–The
  Complete List to enjoy, 154;
  Combined Elimination Diet and
  Kapha Dosha Food List, 173, 175;
  Combined Elimination Diet and
  Pitta Dosha Food List, 169, 171;
  Combined Elimination Diet and Vata
  Dosha Food List, 165, 167

constipation, 71–72

cravings: Ayurvedic herbs will help
  control, 91; as enemy of the CLEAN7
  program, 70

creatinine, 14

Creative Visualization (Gawain), 110

cryotherapy, 77

CSA (Community Sponsored
  Agriculture), 64

Csikszentmihalyi, Mihaly, 112, 113

D

dairy and egg products: CLEAN Diet–
  foods to avoid, 155; Combined
  Elimination Diet and Pitta
  Dosha Food List, 170; Combined
  Elimination Diet and Vata Dosha
  Food List, 164, 166; Elimination
  Diet avoidance of, 142; Kapha Dosha
  Food List, 162, 163; Pitta Dosha Food
  List, 160; pre-cleanse yourself of, 76;
  Vata Dosha Food List, 158, 159

dairy substitutes: CLEAN Diet, 154;
  Combined Elimination Diet and
  Kapha Dosha Food List, 172, 174;
  Combined Elimination Diet and
  Pitta Dosha Food List, 168

Day 1 of CLEAN7, 85–87, 141, 146

Day 2 of CLEAN7, 89, 141, 147

Day 3 of CLEAN7, 92, 141, 148

Day 4 of CLEAN7, 95, 141, 149

Day 5 of CLEAN7, 97, 141, 150

Day 6 of CLEAN7, 101–2, 141, 151

Day 7 of CLEAN7, 103, 141, 152

DDT pesticides, 18

decongestants, 18

deep sleep, 81

depression: author's experience with,
  24, 108–10, 134; how meditation
  helps negativity and, 114–18

"detox blind," 9

detoxification: as ancient medical
  tradition, 12–13, 20; at The We
  Care Spa (Palm Springs), 24, 45–46;
  Ayurvedic herbs used for, 44–45;
  Ayurvedic Medicine's practice of,
  13, 20, 36; basic concepts and
  benefits of, 3–11; CLEAN7 follow-up
  with periodic, 177–78; Functional
  Medicine's focus on, 25–26; the good
  news about, 20–21; intermittent
  fasting benefits for, 51–52; meditation
  for mental and emotional, 84, 96–98;
  mislabeled as "celebrity fad," 10;
  problems which may affect results
  of, 100–101; understanding what
  it means, 13–14. *See also* the body;
  CLEAN7 program; toxicity

Detoxifier Shake recipe: kapha recipe,
  253–54; pitta body type, 226–27;
  vata body type, 201–2

detoxing homes: eliminating toxic air
  offenders, 180; HEPA filters, 180–81;
  importance of air, 179–80; online
  resources on, 183; purifying your
  air, 180–81; water filtration systems,
  182–83. *See also* toxicity

diabetes: as consideration for CLEAN7 program, 57; hypoglycemia and, 53; sleep deprivation associated with, 103

diethanolamine (DEA), 17

diets: Atkins, 12; fat-lowing, 12; keto, 12, 48; low-carb, 12; paleo, 12; pre-cleanse, 76–77. *See also* Elimination Diet (ED)

dinners, historic evolution of breakfast, lunch, and, 50–51

The Dirty Dozen, 64, 66

dosha charts: Chart 1–Vata Dosha Food List, 158–59; Chart 2–Pitta Dosha Food List, 160–61; Chart 3–Kapha Dosha Food List, 162–63; Chart 4–Combined Elimination Diet and Vata Dosha Food List, 164–67; Chart 5–Combined Elimination Diet and Pitta Dosha, 168–71; Chart 6–Combined Elimination Diet and Kapha Dosha Food List, 172–75

doshas system: Ayurvedic thinking on the body types of, 38–40; bidoshic doshas, 60; CLEAN7 application of the, 40–41; CLEAN7 recipes to fit specific, 60; determine your Ayurvedic dosha, 59–61; get the most out of CLEAN7 recipes by using, 187–88; kapha (predominance of earth and water), 38, 39, 157, 162–63, 172–75, 245–71; kapha-vata, 39; pitta (predominance of fire and water), 38, 39, 157, 160–61, 220–44; pitta-kapha, 39; prakriti (primordial dosha type), 41–42, 60, 61; tridoshic doshas, 39, 60; vata (predominance of fire and water), 38, 39, 156, 158–59, 164–67, 194–219; vata-pitta, 39; vikriti (momentary dosha imbalance), 39, 60, 61. *See also* the body

Dr. Schulze's Intestinal Formula #1, 72

dysbiosis, 31

E

eating late tip, 90

eating patterns: breakfast, lunch, and dinner, 50–51; evolution and disruption of feasting and fasting, 46–50

eclectic medicine, 43

eczema, 132

eggplants: as Clean Fifteen food, 67; pre-cleanse yourself of, 77

eggs. *See* dairy and egg products

Ehret, Arnold, 46

elastic band exercise, 111

Elimination Diet (ED): CLEAN7 diet as the personalization of the, 142; to eliminate common dietary triggers, 27; the Five Rs used with, 29–31; as Functional Medicine tool, 177; introduction to the, 27–29; pre-cleanse, 76–77. *See also* diets

Elimination Diet Food Lists: Chart 4–Combined Elimination Diet and Vata Dosha Food List, 164–67; Chart 5-Combined Elimination Diet and Pitta Dosha, 168–71; Chart 6–Combined Elimination Diet and Kapha Dosha Food List, 172–75

emotions: CLEAN7 benefits for calming, 78–79; toxicity and irritability, 73

endocrine disrupters, 17, 18

endogenous toxins, 13–14

enemas, 84, 91–93

energy: CLEAN7 and increased, 80; intermittent fasting and

increased, 55; *The Law of Attraction* on phenomena of, 110; negative thoughts draining, 108

Environmental Working Group, 64, 179

enzymatic reactions: detoxification and, 20; glucuronidation, 20; methylation, 20; sulfation, 20

equanimity, 78–79

erectile dysfunction meds, 17

essential fatty acids, 30

ethylene, 17

exercise/movement: as boosting your CLEAN7 program, 84, 94–96; to help constipation, 72; to help with headaches, 73; meditation exercises, 116–22; reaching state of flow, 112–13; running, 112; yoga, 7, 72, 73

Expedite, Saint, 32

F

Fakora recipe: kapha body type, 270–71; pitta body type, 243–44; vata body type, 218–19

Farzad (friend), 80

Fasting and Easting for Health (Fuhrman), 46

fasting. *See* intermittent fasting

fat-loving diets, 12

FD&C red #40, 19

fear, 16–17

female hormones: disrupters of, 17, 18; shatavari, moringa, and brahmi balancing, 61

fiber, CLEAN7 recipes providing, 30

fight-or-flight reaction, 110, 111, 113

fish. *See* animal/fish protein

the Five Rs: *Reinoculate,* 31; *Relax,* 31; *Remove,* 29–30; *Repair,* 30; *Restore,* 30

Flint, Michigan, water contamination, 181

Flow (Csikszentmihalyi), 112, 113

flow state, 112–13

food allergy tests, 9, 27–28

Food and Drug Administration (FDA), 11

food labels: USDA 100 percent Organic, 65; USDA Organic, 65

food lists: to avoid during state of balance or imbalance, 39–40; Chart 1–Vata Dosha Food List, 158–59; Chart 2–Pitta Dosha Food List, 160–61; Chart 3–Kapha Dosha Food List, 161–63; Chart 4–Combined Elimination Diet and Vata Dosha, 164–67; Chart 5–Combined Elimination Diet and Pitta Dosha, 168–71; Chart 6–Combined Elimination Diet and Kapha Dosha, 168–71; CLEAN Diet–The Complete List to avoid, 155; The Clean Fifteen, 64, 67; The Dirty Dozen, 64, 66

food processors, 62, 190–91

foods: eliminating toxic, 63; gaining an understanding of, 9; "heating," 40; irradiated, 65, 66; organic, 65–66; vata-aggravating, 39; whole, 63–65

Francis, Drew, 24–25

fruits: CLEAN Diet–foods to avoid, 155; CLEAN Diet–The Complete List to enjoy, 154; Combined Elimination Diet and Kapha Dosha Food List, 172, 174; Combined Elimination Diet and Pitta Dosha Food List, 168, 170; Combined Elimination Diet and Vata Dosha Food List, 164, 166; Kapha Dosha Food List, 162, 163;

fruits (*continued*)
  Pitta Dosha Food List, 160, 161; Vata
  Dosha Food List, 158, 159
Fuhrman, Dr. Joel, 46
fun activities, 31
Functional Medicine: AFMCP course
  on, 25–26; author's study of, 22–26;
  Ayurvedic principles within, 133–34;
  CLEAN7 based on principles of, 7–8,
  20, 26–31, 36; combining ancient
  knowledge and modern science,
  13; empowering the body to reach
  healing potential, 30; meaning of
  detoxification in, 14; on mind-body
  connection, 31; systems approach
  of, 20. *See also* CLEAN7 program;
  medicine
Functional Medicine practitioners,
  57, 177
Functional Medicine principles:
  The Elimination Diet, 27–29; the
  Five Rs (Remove, Restore, Repair,
  Reinoculate, Relax), 29–31

G
gallstones, 100
Gawain, Shakti, 110
gene research, 8
Genexa, 18, 19
glucuronidation, 20
glutamine, 30
gluten elimination, 100
glyphosate, 18
GMOs, 63
Golden Cabinet, 24
gout, 100
grains: to avoid, 155; CLEAN diet
  starch/non-gluten grains, 154;
  Combined Elimination Diet and
  Kapha Dosha Food List, 172, 174;
  Combined Elimination Diet and
  Pitta Dosha Food List, 168, 170;
  Combined Elimination Diet and Vata
  Dosha Food List, 164, 166; Kapha
  Dosha Food List, 162, 163; Pitta
  Dosha Food List, 160, 161;
  Vata Dosha Food List, 158, 159
grapefruit, pre-cleanse yourself of, 76
grapes, as Dirty Dozen food, 66
Greco-Arabic medicine, 43
Greek Salad recipe, 276–77
Guide to Reintroduction, of toxic foods
  or triggers, 139
gut permeability, *Repair* (the Five Rs)
  to reduce, 30

H
habit formation, 106–7
headaches, 72–73
healing practices: detoxification, 3–4;
  Functional Medicine empowering
  the body for, 30; by Jesus, 32; power
  of intermittent fasting, 48–49, 51–52,
  54–55
health: author's experience with
  recovering his, 2–5, 23–26, 108–16;
  why do people get sick?, 2
heart disease, 103
"heating" foods, 40
heavy metal toxicity, 100
HEPA filters, 18–181
herbal supplements. *See* Ayurvedic
  herbs
Hicks, Abraham, 110
Hicks, Esther, 110
high fructose corn syrup, 19
honeydew melons, as Clean Fifteen
  food, 67
hormone disrupters, 17, 18
hot and cold plunges, 84, 88–90

hunger, 69–70
hyperpermeability. *See* leaky gut
hypertension, 103
hypoglycemic, 53
Hypromellose, 19

I

IBS (irritable bowel syndrome), 24, 134
I Had to Survive (Canessa), 23
illnesses. *See* sickness/illnesses
imagining technique, 110
immune system, 79–80
impatience, 73–74
Implant-O-Rama, 72, 91
India: Ayurvedic herbs found in
    "go-downs" in, 126; the "green
    revolution" impact on, 126–27;
    reviving the Azamgath village
    in, 129–31; suicide rate of farmers
    in, 127
Indian Vedic nutrition, 42–43
Instapot, 62
insulin: Ayurvedic herbs will help
    regulate, 91; feasting and surge of,
    47; hypoglycemia after too much, 53
intermittent fasting: barriers to, 52–54;
    CLEAN7 based on principles of, 7, 8,
    54–55; defining fasting and, 51–52;
    follow CLEAN7 with regular, 177;
    healing power of, 48–49, 51–52, 54–
    55; lack of scientific understanding
    of, 21; medical role in Germany,
    46; nature's design of intermittent
    feasting and, 46–50; religious-based,
    45, 53. *See also* CLEAN7 program
International Institute for Herbal
    Medicine, 128
intestines: detoxification effect on the,
    25; dysbiosis and hyperpermeability
    (leaky gut), 31; immune system

located within, 79–80; *Reinoculate*
    with good bacteria, 31; *Remove* to
    remove harmful bacteria from,
    29–30
irradiated foods, 65, 66
irritability, 73
irritable bowel syndrome (IBS), 24, 134
Island Strong Shake recipe: kapha
    recipe, 246; pitta body type, 221;
    vata body type, 195

J

Jackman, Hugh, 54
Jagger, Mick, 26
Japanese Traditional Medicine
    (Kampo), 43
Jesus Christ, 32, 45
Jourdan, Pablo, 32
journaling, 67–68, 102, 105

K

Kampo (Japanese Traditional
    Medicine), 43
kapha body type: Combined
    Elimination Diet and Kapha Dosha
    Food List, 172–75; identifying your,
    38, 39, 157; Kapha Dosha Food List,
    162–63
kapha recipes: meals and snacks,
    256–71; shakes, 245–55
kapha-vata dosha, 39
keto diet, 12, 48
ketosis, 48
kidneys: Ayurvedic Medication healing
    the, 132; creatinine used to measure
    function of, 14; detoxification effect
    on the, 25
King George's Medical University, 128
King Kullen (New York City
    supermarket), 49

Kitchari recipe: kapha recipe, 259–60; pitta body type, 233–34; vata body type, 207–8

kitchen: countertop appliances to have, 62–63, 188–91; preparing for CLEAN7 program, 62–63

kiwis, as Clean Fifteen food, 67

L

The Law of Attraction (Hicks and Hicks), 110

laxatives, 72

lead, 17

leaky gut, 31

Lee, Dr., 33

Lemon Vinaigrette recipe: Greek Salad, 276–77; kapha recipe, 264; vata body type, 212

Lenox Hill Hospital (Manhattan), 23, 109

Lent fasting, 45

Lime Vinaigrette recipe, 237–38

liquid meals: CLEAN7 tip on eating late, 90, 92–93; CLEAN7 tip on making shakes, 87, 93; Day 1 of CLEAN7, 85–87, 141; Day 2 of CLEAN7, 89, 141; Day 3 of CLEAN7, 92, 141; Day 4 of CLEAN7, 95, 141; Day 5 of CLEAN7, 97, 141; Day 6 of CLEAN7, 101–2, 141; designing your personalized CLEAN7, 141; different types of, 89; try dosha-suitable shakes, 93

liver: 30, 88; Ayurveda Medicine treatment of weak, 42; detoxification effect on the, 25

low-carb diets, 12

lunches, historic evolution of breakfast, dinner, and, 50–51

lymphatic massage, 99

lymph nodes, detoxification effect on the, 25

M

magnesium powder, 72, 73

magnesium stearate, 19

mangos, as Clean Fifteen food, 67

Manisha, Dr., 32–35

massage, 73, 99

The Maulana Azad Medical College (New Delhi), 41

meal and snack recipes: celebratory meals, 272–83; for kapha body type, 245–71; for pitta body type, 220–44; for vata body type, 194–219

meals: evolution of breakfast, lunch, and dinner, 50–51; family and social association with, 51; liquid, 89

meats. *See* animal/fish protein

medical research: on intermittent fasting, 8; lacking on intermittent fasting, 21; understanding the fallacies of, 11–12

medications: affected by a detox program, 57; modern lifestyle embracing, 17; over-the-counter, 14, 18–19; taken for chronic issues, 15–16; as traditional approach of psychiatry, 108, 110; treating symptoms instead of healing, 3. *See also* Ayurvedic herbs

medicine: as art restoration, 21; Chinese, 13, 24–25, 43; CLEAN7 unifying modern and ancient, 7, 41–43; Functional Medicine combining modern and ancient, 13. *See also* Ayurvedic Medicine; Functional Medicine meditation: author's experience with, 113–15; calming anxiety and negativity, 114–18; detoxing mentally and emotionally with, 84, 96–98; *Relax* through, 31

meditation exercises: The Anchor, 116–17; The Anchor in Motion, 117–18; Meisner Technique, 119–22

Meisner, Sanford, 119, 121, 122

Meisner Technique, 119–22

mental clarity, 78

mental health: author's experience with depression and, 24, 108–16; the calming power of meditation on, 114–18; depression, 24, 108–10, 114–18, 134; how psychiatry approaches, 108, 110. *See also* sickness/illnesses

metabolism/metabolic rate, 42, 53–54

methylation, 20

micronutrients, 30. *See also* nutrients

mind-body connection, 31

mindful breathing, 104

minerals, 44

Mitra, Bharat, 124–33

Mitra, Bhavani, 124, 126, 129

mixed bed deionization, 182

modern lifestyle, 14–19

monk (ashram clinic patient), 34–35

mood changes, 73

Morbidity and Mortality Weekly Report (2016), 102–3

moringa, 44, 61

movement. *See* exercise/movement

Mucusless Diet Healing System (Ehret), 46

multi-cooker (Instapot), 62, 189–90

muscle mass, 53–54

N

Narendra, Dr. (Singh), 36, 38, 44, 61, 128–35, 181

nature: animals follow the rules of, 1–2, 4, 15; Ayurveda Medicine on healing power of, 33; evolution and disruption of feasting and fasting design, 46–50; healing practices aligning the body with, 4–5; preservation-survival safety feature in, 50

nectarines (Dirty Dozen), 66

negativity: accumulation of ama creating, 33, 36–37, 39–40, 79, 115; author's experience with feeling, 108–14; experiencing bad dreams and, 73; meditation for calming, 114–18

Neighborhood Playhouse (New York City), 119

New York University Downtown Hospital, 23

nightmares, 73

nightshade vegetables, 77

nitrates, 18

Nityananda, Bhagawan, 32

noncompliance, 74

non-gluten grains, 154

nutrients: Ayurvedic herbs providing, 44; CLEAN7 recipes providing all necessary, 30. *See also* micronutrients

nutrition: Ayurvedic principles of, 42–43; Indian Vedic, 42–43. *See also* Ayurvedic herbs

nuts: CLEAN Diet–The Complete List to enjoy, 154; Combined Elimination Diet and Kapha Dosha Food List, 173, 175; Combined Elimination Diet and Pitta Dosha Food List, 169,

nuts (*continued*)
171; Combined Elimination Diet and Vata Dosha Food List, 165, 167; foods to avoid, 155; Kapha Dosha Food List, 163; Pitta Dosha Food List, 160, 161; Vata Dosha Food List, 158

O

obesity: sleep deprivation associated with, 103; weight loss and, 42, 43, 79–80
ochratoxin A, 18
oils: CLEAN Diet–The Complete List to enjoy, 154; Combined Elimination Diet and Kapha Dosha Food List, 173, 175; Combined Elimination Diet and Pitta Dosha Food List, 169, 171; Combined Elimination Diet and Vata Dosha Food List, 165, 167; foods to avoid, 155, 159
onions (Clean Fifteen), 67
Ooey-Gooey Brownies recipe, 283
orange juice pre-cleanse, 76
oranges pre-cleanse, 76
organic foods, 65–66
ORGANIC INDIA: CLEAN's partnership with, 134–35; the origins and development of, 125–31; as recommended brand for Ayurvedic herbs, 62
organochlorine pesticides, 18
over-the-counter medications: Genexa's non-toxic, 18, 19; taken for minor symptoms, 14; toxicity of common, 18–19

P

Pablo (study partner), 45
painkillers, 18

paleo diet, 12
Papaji (guru), 32, 125–26
papayas (Clean Fifteen), 67
parabens, 17
parasites, 100
Parrado, Fernando, 23, 114
PBDEs (polybrominated diphenyl ethers), 180
peaches (Dirty Dozen), 66
peanuts pre-cleanse, 77
pears (Dirty Dozen), 66
peppers pre-cleanse, 77
perchlorate, 18
perchlorethylene (PERC), 17
Persistent Organic Pollutants (POPs), 19
pesticides: The Dirty Dozen treated with, 64, 66; toxicity of, 18
4-phenyicyclohexane (4-PC), 17
phthalates, 17
phytomedicines, 445
pineapples (Clean Fifteen), 67
pitta body type: Combined Elimination Diet and Pitta Dosha, 168–71; identifying your, 38, 39, 157; Pitta Dosha Food List, 160–61; recipes for, 220–44
pitta constitution, 34
pitta-kapha dosha, 39
pitta recipes: meals and snacks, 230–44; shakes, 220–29
planetary body, 134–35
planners, 82
plant medicines, 44
polycystic ovarian syndrome, 43
polyvinyl chloride (PVC), 179–80
"positive thinking," 111
potatoes: as Dirty Dozen food, 66; pre-cleanse yourself of, 77

prakriti (primordial dosha type), 38–42, 60, 61

prana (life force), 44, 128

pre-cleanse diet, 76–77

present/presence: experience of not feeling, 110–11; flow connected to state of, 113; meditation to enter natural state of, 113–15

primitive cultures, 15

processed foods, toxicity of, 17–18

propylene glycol, 17, 19

protein. *See* animal protein; vegetable protein

psychiatry, 108, 110

Q

quantum ama, 115

questionnaires. *See* CLEAN7 questionnaires

Quinoa Tabouleh recipe: kapha body type, 268–69; pitta body type, 241–42; vata body type, 216–17

R

Ramakrishna, 32

Ramana Maharshi, 32

Raspberries and Cream Shake recipe, 273

recipes. *See* CLEAN7 recipes

red blood cells analogy, 135

reflecting, 104–6, 136–38

Refreshing Mojito recipe, 280

Reinoculate (the Five Rs), 31

Relax (the Five Rs), 31

religious-based fasting, 45, 53

remineralization of water, 182

Remove (the Five Rs), 29–30

Repair (the Five Rs), 30

Restore (the Five Rs), 30

rest. *See* sleep and rest

reverse osmosis (RO) membrane, 182

running exercise, 112

Ruskin, John, 119, 122

Ruskin School (Los Angeles), 119

S

Salud Shake recipe: kapha recipe, 255; pitta body type, 228–29; vata body type, 203

the Samhitas, 33

saunas, 77, 84, 88

schizophrenia, 108

sea turtle rescue mission, 1

seeds: CLEAN Diet–The Complete List to enjoy, 154; Combined Elimination Diet and Kapha Dosha Food List, 173, 175; Combined Elimination Diet and Pitta Dosha Food List, 169, 171; Combined Elimination Diet and Vata Dosha Food List, 165, 167; Kapha Dosha Food List, 162, 163; Pitta Dosha Food List, 160, 161; Vata Dosha Food List, 158, 159

setting your intention, 57–58

shake recipes: celebratory, 273; for kapha body type, 245–55; for pitta body types, 220–29; for vata body type, 194–203. *See also* breakfasts

shakes: CLEAN7 tip on doubling your, 87, 93; CLEAN7 tip on eating late, 90, 92–93; designing your personalized CLEAN7, 141; liquid meal out of, 89; one every day, 176; trying dosha-suitable, 93

Sharma, Dr. Shikha, 41–43

shatavari, 61

shellfish pre-cleanse, 77

Shirdi Sai Baba, 32

The Shocking Truth About Water (Bragg), 181
shrimp: pre-cleanse yourself of, 77; Vata Dosha Food List, 158
sickness/illnesses: author's story on finding answers to, 2–5, 23–26, 108–16; medications taken for chronic, 15–16; modern lifestyle and stresses causing, 14–19; why do people get sick?, 2. *See also* mental health
Singh, Dr. Narendra, 36, 38, 44, 61, 128–35, 181
Singh, Kailash Nath, 130, 131
skin brushing, 100
sleep and rest: bad dreams, 73; booster of, 102–4; CDC study (2016) on, 102–3; CLEAN7 and deeper, 81; ridding body of toxicity during, 17
smoothies: designing your personalized CLEAN7, 141; liquid meal out of, 89
snacking: helpful suggestions on, 90–91; suggestions for types of healthy, 69–70
snack recipes: pitta body type meal and, 230–44; vata body type meal and, 204–19
soaking practices, 188
social pressure, 71
sodium erythorbate nitrosamines, 18
sodium lauryl sulfate (SLS), 17
Soother Shake recipe: kapha recipe, 247–48; pitta body type, 222; vata body type, 196
soups: designing your personalized CLEAN7, 141; liquid meal out of, 89
soybeans/soy products: foods to avoid, 155; pre-cleanse yourself of, 77
spinach (Dirty Dozen), 66

sports massage, 99
starch/non-gluten grains, 154
state of flow, 112–13
Steven (friend), 124
strawberries (Dirty Dozen), 66
stress: detoxing quantum toxins of, 73; modern lifestyle and, 14–19
stretching exercises, 72, 73
Stuffed Mushrooms recipe, 278–79
sucralose, 19
sugar: foods to avoid, 155; headaches and, 72; possible responses by body to eliminating, 100; pre-cleanse yourself of, 76; sweeteners to use instead of, 154; tips on controlling craving for, 91. *See also* sweeteners
sulfation, 20
sweating, 87–88
Swedish massage, 99
sweet bell peppers (Dirty Dozen), 66
sweet corn (Clean Fifteen), 67
sweeteners: CLEAN Diet–The Complete List to enjoy, 154; Combined Elimination Diet and Kapha Dosha Food List, 173, 175; Combined Elimination Diet and Pitta Dosha Food List, 169, 171; Combined Elimination Diet and Vata Dosha Food List, 165, 167. *See also* sugar
Sweet Mustard Salmon recipe, 281–82
sweet peas (Clean Fifteen), 67
Sweet Potato Hash recipe, 274–75
symptom treating, 14

T
Textbook of Functional Medicine (Baker and others), 26
Tibetan medicine, 43

Tiger's Milk Shake recipe: kapha recipe, 249–50; pita recipe, 223; vata body type, 197–98

Tom (ashram clinic nurse), 33

tomatoes: as Dirty Dozen food, 66; pre-cleanse yourself of, 77

toxic foods: The Clean Fifteen, 64, 67; eliminating, 63; Guide to Reintroduction, 139

toxicity: CLEAN7 protocol to reduce your body's, 65; of the contemporary household, 179–80; cumulative effect of, 19–20; Functional Medicine addressing overload of, 7–8; heavy metal, 100; mislabeled as "celebrity fad" concept, 10; of modern lifestyle, 14–19; traditional poisoning meaning of, 13. *See also* detoxification; detoxing homes

toxins/carcinogens: ama, 33, 36–37, 39–40, 79, 115; creatinine, 14; endogenous, 13–14, 18; modern lifestyle exposure to, 17–20

tridoshic doshas, 39, 60

triethanolamine (TEA), 17

trigger point massage, 99

trihalomethanes (THMs), 17

triphala, 44, 61

tulsi (holy basil), 44, 61–62, 130

tulsi tea, 61–62, 102

turmeric, 44, 61

Tur-Veggie Patty recipe: kapha recipe, 263–65; pitta body type, 237–38; vata body type, 211–12

type 1 diabetes, 53, 57

U

undetected parasites, 100

USDA 100 percent Organic, 65

USDA Organic, 65

V

vacation time, 31

vata-aggravating foods, 39

"vata attack," 39

vata body type: Combined Elimination Diet and Vata Dosha Food List, 164–67; identifying your, 38, 39, 156; recipes for, 194–219; vata-aggravating foods for, 39; Vata Dosha Food List, 158–59

vata-pitta dosha, 39

vata recipes: meals and snacks, 204–19; shakes, 194–203

the Vedas, 33

vegetable protein: Clean Diet–foods to enjoy, 154; Combined Elimination Diet and Kapha Dosha Food List, 173, 175; Combined Elimination Diet and Pitta Dosha Food List, 169, 171; Combined Elimination Diet and Vata Dosha Food List, 164, 167

vegetables: CLEAN Diet–The Complete List to enjoy, 154; Combined Elimination Diet and Kapha Dosha Food List, 172, 174; Combined Elimination Diet and Pitta Dosha Food List, 168, 170; Combined Elimination Diet and Vata Dosha Food List, 164, 166; Kapha Dosha Food List, 162, 163; nightshade, 77; Pitta Dosha Food List, 160, 161; Vata Dosha Food List, 158, 159

Veronica (ashram clinic patient), 33–34

vikriti (momentary dosha imbalance): description of, 39; questionnaire to reveal your, 39–42, 60, 61, 142

visualization technique, 110

W

Waffle Hash Open-Face Sandwich
    recipe: kapha recipe, 261–62;
    pitta body type, 235–36;
    vata body type, 209–10
water contamination, 181–82
water filtration systems, 182–83
We Care Spa (Desert Hot Springs),
    24, 45–46
weight loss, 42, 43, 54, 79–80
"wellness paralysis," 8
Wendling, William, 181–83
whole foods: defining, 63–64;
    where to purchase, 64–65
Whole Foods Market, 62
Wolverine (film), 54

X

xenobiotics, 14

Y

yoga, 7, 72, 73
Yogananda, Paramahansa, 32
Yom Kippur fasting, 45

Z

zinc, 30